Spinal Stenosis:

Understanding the Problem and Finding the Best Solutions For Symptom Relief

Dr. George Best, D.C.

Table of Contents

Disclaimer and Additional Resources..1

Chapter 1: What Is Spinal Stenosis? 2

Types of Spinal Stenosis 2

    Cervical Spine Versus Lumbar Spine...5

    Causes of Acquired Stenosis 6

Chapter 2: Diagnosing Spinal Stenosis..11

Symptoms and Examination Findings...11

Diagnostic Imaging and Other Tests 12

Chapter 3: Symptom Severity Versus Condition Severity 15

Pain Versus Numbness 15

Symptom Severity and Recovery 15

Chapter 4: Talking With Your Doctor..17

    Where is the stenosis? 17

    What is causing the stenosis? 17

    How severe is the stenosis and the problem(s) causing it?............17

    Is there any other problem contributing to my symptoms? 18

    Is there anything that will likely make it worse?...........................18

Setting Expectations 18

Chapter 5: Self Treatment 20

Chapter 6: Using Cold and Heat..22

Using Cold Packs 22

What About Heat? 23

Chapter 7: Oral Anti-Inflammatories 24

Natural Anti-Inflammatories 24

Chapter 8: Acupressure 26

Cervical Spinal Stenosis Acupressure Points 27

Lumbar Spinal Stenosis Acupressure Points 32

Chapter 9:   Magnets 35

Chapter 10: Orthotics 37

Chapter 11: "Energy Medicine" Techniques 39

Energy Medicine For Physical Pain Relief 39

Energy Medicine for Emotional Stress Management (EFT): 42

Points For Emotional Freedom Technique 44

Chapter 12: Exercises 48

Exercises For Cervical Spine Stenosis: 48

The McKenzie Method for the Cervical Spine 48

Cervical Flexibility and Alignment Exercises....................61

Exercises For Lumbar Spine Stenosis: 66

The McKenzie Method 66

Lumbosacral / Hip Flexibility and Alignment....................73

Low Back Stabilization 76

Chapter 13: Inversion / Home Traction 81

Inversion Devices 81

Not Recommended: Inversion Boots..................................82

Home Traction Devices: 83

Chapter 14: Lifestyle Modifications 86

Diet: 86

Avoid Smoking: 87

Hydration: 88

Activity/General Exercise: 88

Chapter 15: Professional Treatment Options 90

A Word About Health Care Providers 90

Non-Invasive Treatments 91

Spinal Manipulation 91

Massage 92

Physical Therapy 92

Portable Electrical Stimulators 94

Acupuncture 95

Spinal Decompression 96

Oral Prescription Medication 97

Invasive Treatments 98

Injections 98

Surgery 100

Conclusion 105

Review and Connect 106

Disclaimer and Additional Resources

Every case is different and this book is not a substitute for professional evaluation and treatment. Some individuals may require different and/or additional treatments to the ones presented in this book. Readers are advised to pay close attention to the warnings and precautions that are included in this book and are advised to seek medical attention in the event that symptoms worsen or if new symptoms arise.

Further information is available through the author's website at:

http://www.AskDrBest.com/spinal-stenosis-book-resources

Chapter 1: What Is Spinal Stenosis?

The word stenosis means narrowing. In the case of cardiac stenosis, the narrowing is of the blood vessels in the heart. In the case of spinal stenosis, the narrowing is of one or more of the passageways in the spine that the spinal cord and nerves pass through. Spinal stenosis can occur anywhere in the spine, but symptomatic cases tend to be in the mid to lower lumbar spine (in the low back) and in the mid to lower cervical spine (in the neck), and this book will be concentrating on those areas.

Although the term spinal stenosis is often used as a stand alone diagnosis by doctors, it really is quite vague in terms of describing the condition of a given individual. It is this author's opinion that further description is necessary in order to understand the nature and severity of the problem in a given case, and also to know what treatment methods are likely to be most effective for that person.

Types of Spinal Stenosis

There are two main types of spinal stenosis: congenital and acquired. Congenital spinal stenosis is something an individual is born with. In most cases it is a situation in which the pedicles (bony structures that connect the weight-bearing body of each spinal bone to the vertebral arch) of one or more spinal bones are shorter than normal, resulting in a narrower central spinal canal which houses the spinal cord. This is illustrated below:

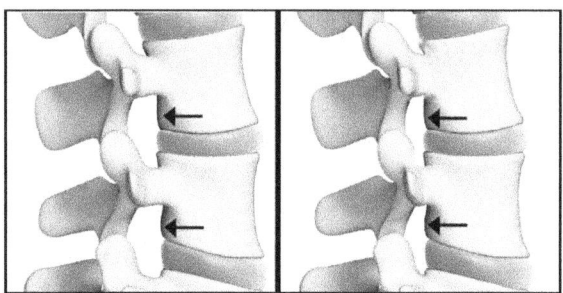

Congenital Stenosis: The image on the left shows a normal section of the spine, while the image on the right shows congenital stenosis. The arrows point to the space where the spinal cord and nerves are located. Notice the decreased spaces in the image on the right.

Congenital stenosis in and of itself rarely causes symptoms, but it does make one more susceptible to the effects of the various causes of acquired stenosis and other conditions of the spine, simply because there is less space in the spinal canal to accommodate other sources of narrowing and increased pressure.

Acquired stenosis refers to any kind of narrowing of the spinal passageways that a person was not born with. There are several common causes of acquired stenosis, and the nature and severity of the cause will have a significant effect on symptoms and will usually help determine what treatment(s) are likely to be most effective in a given case. The common causes of acquired stenosis will be discussed in detail later in this chapter.

Besides the basic type of spinal stenosis, there is also a question of the location of the stenosis in the part of the spine affected, that is, what passageway(s) are narrowed. There are two main passageways that can be involved. The first is known as the central spinal canal which, as was mentioned earlier, houses the spinal cord. The other potential site for stenosis is the intervertebral foramina, which are the openings on both sides of the spine where the spinal nerves branch off from the spinal cord and exit the spine to supply the various muscles, organs, and tissues of the body.

Technically, the term spinal stenosis is generally considered to refer to narrowing of the central spinal canal (also called central stenosis). The term intervertebral stenosis is more correct for describing narrowing of the intervertebral foramina. Intervertebral stenosis also goes by the name foraminal stenosis or lateral stenosis (although there are technically some subtle distinctions between foraminal and lateral stenosis, the causes and treatments are essentially the same and therefore they will be considered the same for the purposes of this book).

Despite the different locations of narrowing, many doctors and healthcare providers simply lump everything together under the term spinal stenosis, and this can sometimes be disadvantageous with regards to deciding on appropriate treatment. From this point forward in this book, the terms central stenosis and intervertebral stenosis will be used when appropriate to distinguish between the two locations of narrowing. The illustrations that follow show the different sites of stenosis in the spine:

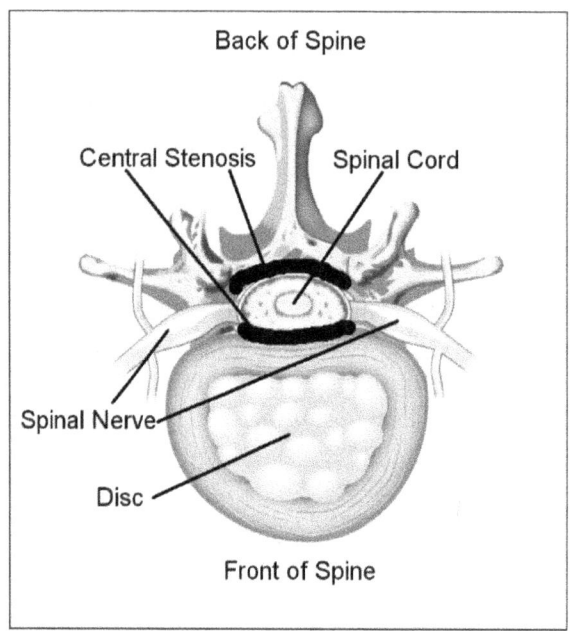

Central Stenosis: *The passageway for the spinal cord is narrowed (as indicated by the thick black lines).*

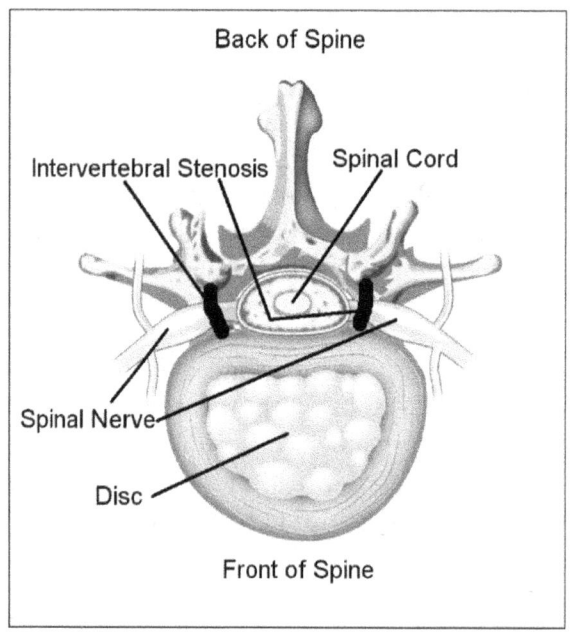

Intervertebral Stenosis: *Narrowing of the openings around one or both spinal nerves (as indicated by the black lines).*

Cervical Spine Versus Lumbar Spine

As stated earlier, the primary sites for spinal stenosis are the lumbar and cervical spinal regions. Central stenosis is somewhat more common in the lumbar spine than the cervical, but cervical cases tend to be more severe symptomatically. This is partly because the central spinal canal is much smaller in diameter in the cervical spine than in the lumbar, and there's less space around the spinal cord for it to shift away from whatever is causing the narrowing. In addition, the spinal cord actually ends about midway down the lumbar spine and becomes a collection of smaller, individual nerve fibers known as the cauda equina (a Latin term meaning "horse's tail", which is descriptive of its appearance). This transition from cord to individual nerve fibers provides a greater ability for the neurological structures to shift and compensate for narrowing of the canal. Since the end of the spinal cord is above the most common area for significant central canal stenosis in the lumbar spine, the potential for serious symptoms from central stenosis is much lower in the low back than it is in the neck.

Because central stenosis in the cervical spine has significant potential to compress the spinal cord and produce progressive damage and interference with its function (you may see the term myelopathy to describe this type of damage to the spinal cord), it can produce symptoms in the neck, arms and/or legs. When central stenosis of the lumbar spine is severe enough to produce symptoms, they are primarily in the legs and/or low back. This can lead to confusion even among doctors, as there is a tendency to assume that neurological symptoms in the legs are always coming from the lumbar spine. The author has seen more than one case over the years in which a patient with leg symptoms stemming from cervical stenosis was treated by their doctor as a malingerer (someone faking symptoms for the purposes of an insurance or legal claim) or a "head case" when no problems could be detected in the lumbar spine.

As opposed to central stenosis, intervertebral stenosis in the lumbar spine tends to produce more severe symptoms than in the cervical spine. Because of the much greater weight that the lumbar spine has to carry, the spinal structures in the low back are much larger than in the cervical spine. When something goes wrong with one or more of the structures associated with intervertebral stenosis, it tends to go more wrong in the lumbar spine than the cervical spine.

Unlike central stenosis in the cervical spine, intervertebral stenosis in the neck is not associated with leg symptoms, but symptoms in the arm, neck, and mid back are common. Lumbar intervertebral stenosis can cause symptoms in the low back, buttock, and/or leg on the side of stenosis. Although intervertebral stenosis is most commonly one-sided, it is possible to have significant stenosis of both intervertebral foramina and therefore have symptoms on both sides.

Causes of Acquired Stenosis

Several underlying issues can cause either or both central and intervertebral stenosis, and it is this author's opinion that it is often more useful to describe the cause of the narrowing rather than, or at least in combination with, using a vague diagnostic term like stenosis. For example, one common cause of central and/or intervertebral stenosis is a disc protrusion. While most health care providers will provide a diagnosis that includes the disc protrusion, I have seen a number of patients with disc protrusions who were told and were given documentation that they had "spinal stenosis" without any further description. This lack of descriptiveness often results in misconceptions by the patients and sometimes even their health care providers as to the nature of their condition and how best to proceed with treatment. This will be explained further as we discuss the various causes in this chapter, and again later in the book when treatment options are covered.

As was just mentioned, a disc protrusion is a common cause of central and/or intervertebral stenosis. The spinal discs are soft tissue structures that provide flexibility and shock absorption to the spine. A spinal disc has an outer wall known as the annulus fibrosis, which is composed of cartilage fibers that surround an inner gel-like core called the nucleus pulposis. Under normal conditions, the outer border of the disc conforms to the border of the vertebral body above and below it. Damage to the disc from trauma, improper lifting, or abnormal wear and tear and degeneration from things such as poor posture, excessive sitting, and other factors can weaken, overstretch, and/or tear the wall of the disc, and the pressure on the inner gel causes an outward bulge at the site of the damage, as in the illustration that follows:

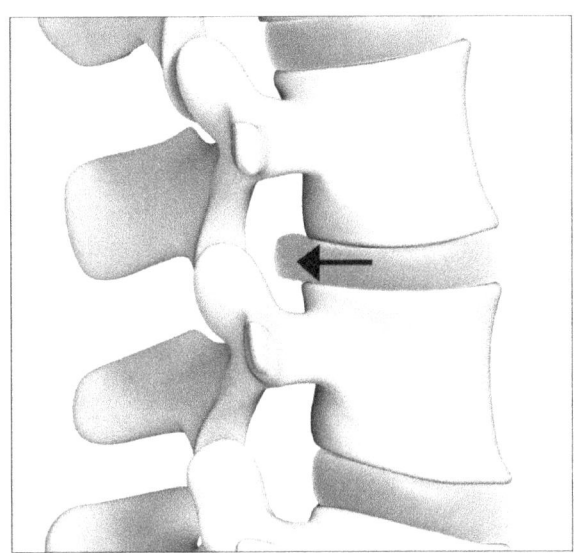

A Disc Protrusion or Herniated Disc

Disc protrusions go by a variety of names, including disc herniations, disc prolapses, disc bulges, or HNPs (Herniated Nucleus Pulposis). Some doctors make distinctions on what they call a disc protrusion based on the severity and/or shape of the protrusion, but unfortunately there is not a universally agreed upon terminology and the varied terms used for what is essentially the same thing can create a lot of confusion for patients. For example, a mild protrusion might be referred to as a bulge, whereas a larger protrusion might be called a herniation. Likewise, a relatively broad-shaped bulge (in which the size of the base is wider than the length) might be called a bulge or herniation, while a more focal bulge (in which the size of the base is about the same or narrower than the length) might be called a protrusion. These distinctions, which vary from doctor to doctor, are not particularly important for patients to know, other than for recognizing the basic meaning of the terminology. Perhaps the most familiar term, "slipped disc", refers to a disc protrusion and not an actual slippage of the disc from between the vertebra as people tend to conceptualize it.

In severe cases of disc herniation, the inner gel of a disc can actually breach the outer wall of the disc. This is called a disc extrusion, or in common terms, a ruptured disc. In some cases of disc extrusions, the gel that has breached the wall is still continuous with the gel remaining inside the disc. In the most severe situations, a quantity of gel may separate from the disc and "float" around in the spinal canals, in which case it is called a sequestrum, or sequestered fragment. Because of the movable nature of a sequestrum, the symptoms associated with it can be extremely variable – severe, crippling symptoms at times and sometimes perhaps no symptoms at all.

It should be noted that the term "ruptured disc" is often used very loosely, even among doctors. In fact, it has been the author's experience that more often than not, the so-called "ruptured" disc is not actually ruptured but is simply bulging. A truly ruptured disc will almost always be designated by the terms extrusion and/or sequestrum/sequestered fragment on imaging reports.

With the exception of most disc extrusions and sequestered fragments, the vast majority of disc issues can be effectively treated and managed without surgery. Specific treatment options will be discussed later in this book.

The other common cause of acquired stenosis, sometimes called "posterior element" stenosis, is actually comprised of some combination of a handful of underlying conditions. These conditions include arthritic spurring, ridging, and/or thickening of the bone surfaces, buckling and/or thickening of the spinal ligaments, and synovial cysts (also called Tarlov cysts) associated with degenerative arthritis in the spinal joints. Posterior element means that the problem is occurring at the back of the spinal canals, whereas a disc protrusion produces narrowing from the front side of the spinal canals.

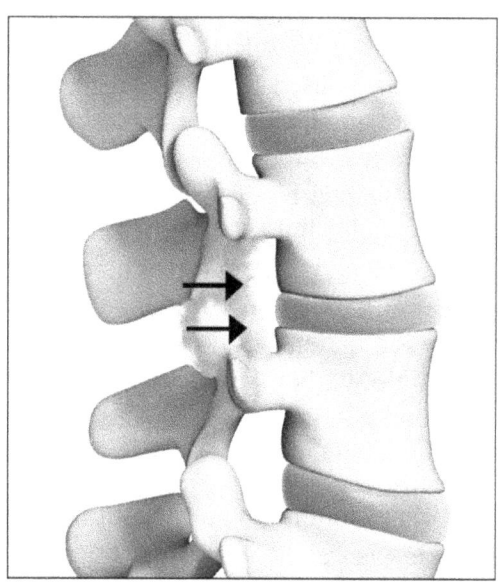

Posterior Element Stenosis: *Narrowing of the back side of the spinal canals, occurring due to degenerative bone formation.*

Bone spurring, ridging, and/or thickening are usually associated with degenerative spinal arthritis and typically occur on and around the facet joints at the back of the spine and/or on the edges of the vertebral body. While the excess bone formation is usually more of a problem when it occurs around the joints at the back of the spine (as part of posterior element stenosis), it can also occur on the back edge of the vertebral body and thereby cause stenosis at the front of the spinal canals as well. When degenerative bone formation occurs in combination with a disc protrusion and/or degeneration, you may see it referred to as a "disc-osteophyte complex" on radiology reports.

Another common potential contributor to posterior element stenosis is thickening and/or buckling of a ligament (called the ligamentum flavum), which runs along the back of the vertebral arches. Thickening and/or buckling of the ligament is commonly seen in association with degenerative disc disease and spinal arthritis. Essentially, as the discs degenerate, they become thinner and the distance between the spinal bones shrinks. The shortened length of the spine in the area of the degenerated disc(s) then results in a ligament that is longer than the span of the spine it covers, and buckling occurs. Loss of disc height also tends to place more mechanical stress on the facet joints and results in degenerative bone formation and ligament thickening, so there is usually some combination of buckling and thickening of the ligament contributing to posterior element stenosis.

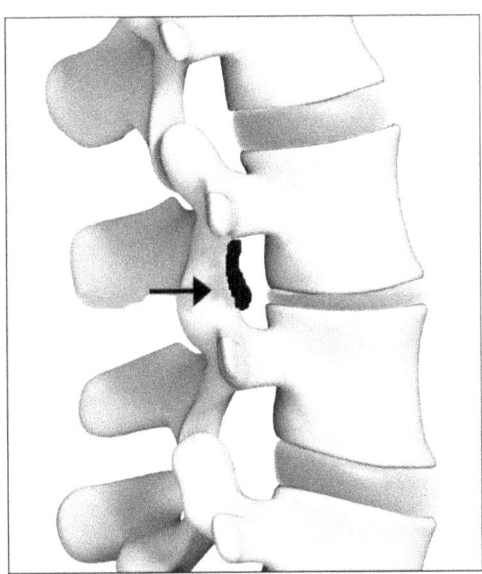

Ligament Thickening and Buckling: *A common result of degenerative disc disease and spinal arthritis.*

Degenerative bone and ligament issues can be more difficult to treat than disc-related stenosis because the tissues involved are less flexible and changeable than discs, but depending on the severity they can still usually be managed with non-surgical methods. This will be discussed further in the section on treatment options.

The last common potential component of posterior element stenosis is synovial cysts, or Tarlov cysts as they are sometimes called. These cysts are primarily seen in cases of arthritis of the spinal facet joints and are most common in the lumbar spine (low back). While not considered dangerous, they can grow large enough to cause significant stenosis by themselves, particularly of the intervertebral foramina (the openings where the nerves exit the spine). Such cysts sometimes shrink on their own, and possibly in response to anti-inflammatory medications. They can be treatment-resistant in some cases; however, and may tend to recur even after surgical removal.

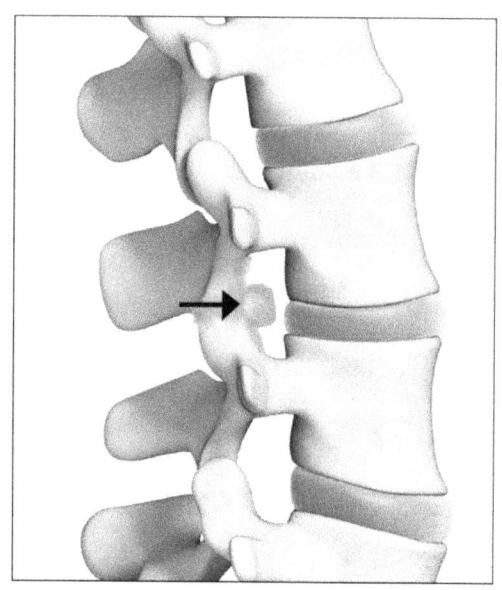

Stenosis Due to Synovial Cyst

Chapter 2: Diagnosing Spinal Stenosis

Since spinal stenosis is not a term that the average person is usually familiar with, chances are if you are reading this book you've had at least some professional evaluation that provided the diagnosis of spinal stenosis. But there are situations in which doctors may make a presumptive diagnosis based on symptoms or, as previously discussed, the vague diagnosis of spinal stenosis may have been provided without further description. Since the specific nature and severity of the condition needs to be understood in order to determine the best treatment options, a discussion of diagnosis is warranted.

Symptoms and Examination Findings

A person's case history and symptoms will often provide big clues as to the nature of the problem. The most noticeable symptoms of spinal stenosis are the result of irritation and/or compression of neurological structures, namely the spinal cord and spinal nerves. Symptoms of spinal cord involvement are somewhat different from the symptoms of spinal nerve involvement, and therefore the types of symptoms a person has may give some information as to whether the stenosis is of the central canal (which tends to produce mainly spinal cord symptoms) or of the intervertebral foramen (which tends to produce primarily spinal nerve symptoms). Bear in mind though that central and intervertebral stenosis can occur together, and this can lead to overlapping symptoms. For this reason, symptoms alone are not a reliable way to definitively diagnose spinal stenosis and further evaluation is required.

The first clue about the location of stenosis is that spinal cord symptoms from central stenosis will often affect both sides of the body relatively symmetrically. Spinal nerve symptoms from intervertebral stenosis are more commonly one-sided, or symptoms will be somewhat different from one side to the other when present on both sides.

Spinal cord (central stenosis) symptoms tend to be more of a loss of sensation (numbness, heaviness, dullness, etc.) and/or impaired control of muscles (weakness, loss of coordination, etc.), rather than pain. Spinal nerve (intervertebral stenosis) symptoms are primarily pain-producing initially, but if the underlying condition is not resolved, the progression of nerve damage over a period of weeks or months will often lead to symptoms more like those associated with the spinal cord (loss of sensation, muscle weakness, etc.).

In long standing and more severe cases, spinal cord compression (central stenosis) may lead to severe loss of muscle function, with the muscles involved becoming very tight and difficult to move (called spastic paralysis). Although intervertebral stenosis usually doesn't progress to the severity where there is significant loss of muscle function, when it does, the damage to the spinal nerves causes the muscles to become very weak and flaccid – essentially the opposite of what occurs with spinal cord compression.

As the evaluation of the patient progresses, another distinguishing characteristic between spinal cord involvement and spinal nerve involvement is found in what are called deep tendon reflexes (when your doctor taps various spots with that little hammer or "tomahawk" and your muscle twitches). Spinal cord issues tend to increase the magnitude of deep tendon reflexes, and can produce reflexes in which the muscle contracts and relaxes multiple times in response to a single tap. Spinal nerve issues will tend to diminish reflexes, making the muscles twitch much less than normal (or not at all) in response to the tap.

Diagnostic Imaging and Other Tests

The direct evaluation of spinal stenosis requires some type of diagnostic imaging. The signs and symptoms discussed up to this point are important to an extent for the direct information they provide, but perhaps are most important for suggesting what type of imaging to do and what part of the body should be imaged. By far the most common imaging continues to be X-rays, although more and more frequently digital X-rays, which are viewed on a computer screen, are replacing the more familiar X-rays produced on large pieces film that have to be placed on a lightbox to be viewed.

X-rays can provide a lot of information about bony or "hard tissue" sources of stenosis, but are usually lacking in information about disc, ligament, and other "soft tissue" problems. An X-ray of the spine only shows the bones in detail. Although some information can be gleaned about the soft tissues, the structures themselves cannot usually be seen in much detail - only the spaces they occupy can be seen clearly. For example X-rays will show disc thinning due to degeneration (because you can see that the space between the spinal bones is reduced), but will give no reliable information on whether the disc is bulging or not.

Since there is often a combination of hard and soft tissue influences on spinal stenosis, X-rays often fail to tell the whole story and can be misleading as to the nature and severity of the problem in a given case. For example, a person with even a fully ruptured disc might have essentially normal X-ray findings. Unfortunately, there still exists a significant number of doctors who are content to stick with X-rays to evaluate their patients, and this can lead to people suffering needlessly for extended periods of time with ineffective and sometimes even counterproductive treatment. The author has even seen some cases where the patient's symptoms were essentially ignored or dismissed as "old age" (or something equally irrelevant to the problem) when X-rays showed no significant abnormalities.

It is this author's opinion that any patient with significant symptoms possibly due to spinal stenosis who is not having much improvement within a few weeks of treatment should be evaluated by MRI or CT scan. These types of scans are far more sensitive than X-rays and will allow visualization of soft tissue structures themselves (not just the spaces they occupy). Of the two, MRI gives a much better diagnostic image of the soft tissues, but it cannot be used in people who have metallic joint replacements or other surgically implanted metal, due to the potentially damaging effects of the large magnetic field of the MRI on them (titanium implants are non-magnetic and do not contraindicate MRI unless combined with other metals). In those cases where MRI cannot be used, CT scans provide a reasonable alternative, but otherwise MRI is the superior imaging option for evaluating possible soft tissue factors in spinal stenosis.

Regardless of the type of imaging done, it is important that the area of evaluation is carefully considered. Here again, the patient's signs and symptoms can help point the doctor in the right direction, but it is easy for even the best of doctors to miss something on the first attempt at diagnosis. As stated earlier, symptoms that might seem to be associated with the lumbar spine can be associated with cervical central canal stenosis. So, although the reasonable first approach might be to perform imaging on the lumbar spine, it may be necessary to take a look at the cervical spine (or even the thoracic spine or other parts of the body) if no significant problems are found in the low back and/or if treatment fails to bring about the desired results.

In addition to advanced imaging, there are various types of neurological tests that can be done to identify the neurological structures involved and the extent of the damage/functional abnormality present. Most often, such tests are performed by, or under the supervision of, a neurologist. Electromyography (EMG) and Nerve Conduction Velocity (NCV) are the most commonly-used tests of this type and they measure the electrical activity of the nerves. These tests are most often done to help pinpoint the problem when imaging and other examination findings are unclear and/or to monitor the patient's progress.

Most doctors are very good about evaluating further when at first getting a conclusive diagnosis and/or positive treatment results is elusive, but some are not and may require some coaxing from you (or a change of doctors). In the author's experience, patients who need something more from a doctor who may be resistant to do more, tend to have a better chance of getting what they need through subtle persuasion than by making demands.

In other words, if you're not improving and you want your doctor to order an MRI or refer you to a specialist, it often works better to ask your doctor questions that lead him or her down the path rather than outright saying, "I want you to send me for an MRI." Sticking with the MRI example, if your doctor only did X-rays and hasn't mentioned doing an MRI, you might say something like, "My friend had symptoms like mine that turned out to be from a cyst that didn't show up on his X-rays. They found it with an MRI. Do you think I might need one?" I know this may seem silly (probably because it is), but for some reason, certain doctors are much more motivated to order tests and referrals when they think it's their idea and not yours.

Chapter 3: Symptom Severity Versus Condition Severity

Patients and even doctors sometimes confuse the nature and/or severity of symptoms with the severity of the underlying condition(s) producing those symptoms. It is important to understand that there is essentially NO correlation between the severity of symptoms and the severity or seriousness of the underlying cause. This is true of many health conditions, but it is especially true in the case of spinal stenosis and other symptomatic conditions of the spine.

Pain Versus Numbness

Let's begin with pain versus numbness. Most people would probably choose numbness over pain (at least severe pain), but the reality is, numbness usually indicates a more severe underlying neurological problem than even the worst pain. Numbness, at least in relation to spinal stenosis, is an indication of long-standing and/or relatively severe compression of one or more neurological structures. Furthermore, it indicates a loss of neurological function and that neurological damage is occurring. Neurological structures do not heal as well as most other tissues in the body, so any damage is a serious situation.

Although short-term numbness is not too worrisome, the longer that numbness is present, the greater the chance that permanent damage to the effected neurological structures will occur. Pain may be more unpleasant than numbness, but pain represents nerve irritation and in fact demonstrates that the nerve function is intact. Pain changing to numbness is a bad sign and is an indication that action should be taken without delay to try to avoid further loss of function. On the other hand, numbness switching to pain is actually a good sign in most cases (if perhaps an unpleasant one) that function is returning and the condition is actually improving.

Symptom Severity and Recovery

Although severe pain is unpleasant to go through and can dramatically interfere with one's life, severity is not a reliable indication of what type of treatment is needed, nor how long it will take to recover. The author has seen patients over the years who were literally carried into his office in agonizing pain who walked out pain-free after a 30 minute treatment (after he corrected a relatively minor underlying issue). He has also seen patients with severe underlying conditions that were essentially untreatable by any means who (luckily for them) had only mild symptoms.

The take away from this is that no matter how bad things may feel at this moment, there is still an excellent chance that you can get better and that you can get better without having to endure an invasive surgery or other scary treatment scenario.

Chapter 4: Talking With Your Doctor

Once you have had the necessary diagnostic evaluations, it is important to get certain information from your doctor regarding the specific findings of those evaluations. While it is certainly your doctor's job to manage your case, it is still important for you to have a good understanding of your condition to be able to best utilize the self-treatment recommendations later in this book, as well as to be able to make an informed decision regarding whatever professional treatment recommendations your doctor may provide.

You may already have some ideas as to what questions to ask based on the information that has already been discussed. But to assist you, the following basic questions are suggested:

Where is the stenosis?

You need to know what general part of the spine it is in (cervical, lumbar, etc.) as well as where the narrowing is occurring in the level(s) effected (for example, is it in the central canal and/or the intervertebral foramen and is it on the right and/or left?). It's also helpful to know whether the narrowing is primarily at the anterior (front) portion or posterior (back) part of the central canal and/or intervertebral foramen, or if there is narrowing coming from both anterior and posterior sources.

What is causing the stenosis?

Is the stenosis due to a disc protrusion, bone spurring/thickening, ligament thickening/buckling, cyst, or some combination of them?

How severe is the stenosis and the problem(s) causing it?

Ask your doctor to quantify it as mild, moderate, or severe by the following definitions: Mild means there is narrowing, but probably not enough by itself to cause significant compression or irritation of the spinal cord or nerves (in such cases, inflammatory swelling is often the main cause of symptoms rather than the stenosis itself). Moderate means the narrowing is bad enough that it probably is causing some direct compression or irritation of the spinal cord or nerves. Severe means the narrowing is visibly (on imaging studies) causing significant compression and/or displacement of the spinal cord or nerves.

Is there any other problem contributing to my symptoms?

In many cases, there are complicating factors that may cause otherwise asymptomatic stenosis to create symptoms. For example, anything that increases general inflammation (seasonal allergies, poor diet, smoking, etc.) can increase swelling around the spine and cause more nerve compression. Diabetes and circulation problems can cause nerve degeneration which may mimic or add to stenosis symptoms. Arthritis in one or more joints may also contribute to pain and other symptoms in the areas affected by the stenosis. In any event, it is good to have an idea of anything your doctor does think is an issue so you can take action when indicated to reduce the impact of those complicating factors if possible.

Is there anything that will likely make it worse?

This topic is going to be covered later in the book, but it is always good to have specific recommendations in this regard from a professional who has personally evaluated you. The exercises and other self-treatments covered later are designed to be safe and effective for the vast majority of cases, but if your doctor has advised against any of them, he or she is in a better position to advise you on your particular situation, so it is strongly recommended that you follow your doctor's recommendation unless doing so seems to be making your condition worse.

Setting Expectations

Finally, when talking with your doctor it is important to find out from him or her, what your expectations should be. Depending on your specific circumstances, your maximum recovery could take anywhere from a few days to a year or more. In addition, the condition you will be in at the point of maximum recovery could range from completely normal and able to do all your normal activities without pain or concern, to having residual and/or recurring symptoms of varying severity that may necessitate you altering your activities.

Now, nobody can predict with 100% certainty, and you may be able to greatly exceed your doctor's expectations by diligently following a self-care program (such as the methods in this book), but try to get some idea of what your doctor expects to happen based on his or her experience with cases like yours. It's also helpful to talk to others who have or had the same types of problems you have to find out their experiences (a simple way to do this is to join online forums for people with spinal stenosis). All too often the author has seen patients with long-standing major underlying issues who expected to be back to 100% normal in a day or two, and that can lead to a lot of frustration and disappointment when it doesn't happen.

Chapter 5: Self Treatment

As was just mentioned in the previous chapter, any recommendations from your doctor or other health care professional who has personally evaluated you will take priority over any recommendations that follow in this book. In addition, it is important, if at all possible, to have the answers to the basic questions from Chapter 3 in order to be able to select the most appropriate self-treatment methods for your particular situation.

Although spinal stenosis can affect the thoracic spine, the vast majority of symptomatic cases involve the cervical and/or lumbar spine instead. For this reason, the treatments discussed reference only the cervical and lumbar spine areas. Thoracic spinal stenosis will often respond favorably to the treatments recommended for the cervical and/or lumbar spine; however, so there is good reason to at least try those methods if you happen to have stenosis in the thoracic spine.

The treatments are presented in order of what will usually be the most reliable and easiest to tolerate (when you are having severe symptoms) first. In most cases, the exercises will provide the best lasting improvement in symptoms, but if you find them too painful to do, simply start with the easier treatments first, which are intended for inflammation and pain control.

Not every method presented works for everybody and you need not use every treatment found in this book. In fact, if you find something that it particularly effective for you it is recommended that, at least initially, you spend most of your time and effort on that method. The other methods can be used later on (or not at all) after the worst of your symptoms are resolved to potentially provide additional improvement.

Exercises are usually a critical component to long-term symptom relief and prevention, so it is highly recommended that you begin using the suggested exercises as soon as you can tolerate them.

Finally, before you delve into the various self-treatment methods, there is one important thing to bear in mind:

WARNING

If you have been diagnosed with SEVERE central canal stenosis, you should not attempt any of the exercises/positions demonstrated in this book , nor use traction or inversion without your doctor's approval. Severe central stenosis presents some unique risks and for this reason, all exercises and traction/inversion treatments should be supervised and/or approved by a qualified health care professional.

Chapter 6: Using Cold and Heat

Inflammation plays at least some role in the vast majority of cases of both central and intervertebral stenosis. Even in cases where the actual stenosis is minimal, inflammatory swelling in the area can produce enough pressure on neurological structures to produce major, and even severely debilitating symptoms. For this reason, inflammation control is always an important aspect of self-care.

WARNING

If you have impaired circulation or decreased skin sensitivity due to nerve damage, diabetes, etc., it is best to check with your doctor first before using cold or heat.

Using Cold Packs

Although there are many over the counter medications and natural anti-inflammatory products, by far the most effective and safest means of controlling inflammation without prescription drugs or injections is using cold packs. The basic rule of thumb for cold packs is to apply them for about 10 minutes at a time in smaller body areas like the neck, and 15 to 20 minutes at a time in larger areas like the low back, at a frequency of up to every 2 hours you are awake (while significant symptoms are present). As symptoms improve, the frequency of applying the cold packs can be gradually decreased and they can be discontinued altogether once the symptoms are gone or have reached a stable, tolerable level.

It is important to separate the cold pack from the skin with a thin layer of cloth such as a t-shirt, to avoid skin damage from the cold. It is also important to avoid applying a cold pack on an area that has been recently treated with Theragesic, Icy Hot, Biofreeze, Ben Gay, or any other topical analgesic. It is recommended that you wait until the sensation of the analgesic has completely worn off and that you clean the skin with soap and water to remove any residue of the analgesic before applying the cold pack. Failure to do this could result in hyper-cooling of the skin, leading to irritation or even frostbite. Finally, you should avoid sleeping on an ice pack or exceeding the time recommendations above, as excessive use of ice can actually trigger an inflammatory response.

What About Heat?

Although heat continues to be a popular self-treatment method, it is counterproductive when inflammation is a significant contributor to symptoms. Many people prefer the sensation of heat to cold, and while heat is being applied it does often reduce symptoms due to sedation of the nervous system. Unfortunately, heat tends to keep inflammation going and it can lead to increased symptoms when the heat pack or heating pad is removed, as well as delay recovery in inflammatory conditions. If your symptoms are primarily of stiffness and soreness rather than sharp pain, heat is fine to try, and use if you find it to be helpful, but when in doubt it is best to avoid heat and use cold packs instead. If you do wish to try heat, the same time and frequency recommendations for cold packs hold true: about 10 minutes at a time on small body areas like the neck and 15 to 20 minutes on the low back up to a frequency of every 2 hours while you are awake. As with cold packs, it is strongly recommended that you DO NOT sleep with a heat pack or heating pad.

Chapter 7: Oral Anti-Inflammatories

The most familiar of the anti-inflammatories that can be taken orally are probably the over the counter versions of various NSAIDs (Non-Steroidal Anti-Inflammatory Drugs), such as aspirin, ibuprofen, and naproxen. Although these medications are all chemically similar, one may work better (and/or have fewer side-effects) than another for a given individual. All of these medications can potentially cause gastrointestinal bleeding and other serious side-effects, so it is good to be cautious with their usage. Always follow the dosage recommendations and avoid combining multiple over the counter NSAIDS or combining them with any prescription anti-inflammatories you may be taking.

Although a popular over the counter medication for spinal stenosis and pain in general, Tylenol (Acetaminophen) does not have any anti-inflammatory effects and is strictly a pain-reliever. It has been the author's experience that in most cases, people with symptoms from spinal stenosis will get better results in the long run using anti-inflammatory products rather than Tylenol.

Natural Anti-Inflammatories

WARNING

If you are already taking either over-the-counter or prescription anti-inflammatory medications, or you are on blood-thinning drugs such as Coumadin (warfarin), it is strongly recommended that you consult with a pharmacist or licensed healthcare provider before starting any nutritional anti-inflammatories, as there is a potential for dangerous interactions.

There are many natural anti-inflammatory supplements, but among the most popular and best-documented by scientific research are: omega-3 fatty acids (EPA and DHA – mostly commonly from fish oil, but krill oil or walnut oil are also good sources), bromelain, hesperidin, quercetin, curcumin (turmeric), MSM, ginger, and aloe vera. Omega-3 products tend to be primarily Omega-3 (with perhaps a few other ingredients to stabilize them). Other natural anti-inflammatory products often combine two or more of the other ingredients just mentioned and such combination products can be quite effective.

Homeopathic remedies for reducing pain and inflammation may also be useful, and there are many such remedies. For best results with homeopathy, I recommend consulting with a homeopathic physician to get the remedy that is best suited to your particular needs. Alternately, there are combination formulas available where nutritional supplements are sold. These are usually intended for the general treatment of pain and inflammation and they can often provide good results.

As with medications, different natural anti-inflammatories work better for one person than another. For the sake of simplicity, during times of significant inflammation, I recommend using Omega-3 fatty acids (at a dose that provides approximately 800 - 1,000 mg of EPA per day, which is usually 2000 to 6000 mg of fish oil, depending on the source and purity of the product), and/or a product with a combination of two or more of the other substances mentioned (follow package instructions for dosing recommendations). It is usually beneficial to take at least some omega-3 every day even once symptoms are gone, but the dosage can be cut in half when used for prevention rather than to treat significant inflammation. Ginger can also be eaten in various forms as opposed to being taken as a supplement - some people find candied crystallized ginger an effective and tasty anti-inflammatory.

Chapter 8: Acupressure

Acupressure can be helpful for alleviating symptoms from both nerve compression and muscle contraction forms of sciatica.

Acupressure points can be stimulated by pressing / massaging with your fingers, "pulsing" them with the spring-loaded button of a ball-point pen (see picture that follows), or, if you happen to have a laser pointer available (a red laser with a 630 – 635 nm wavelength is recommended), you can direct the laser on the points as shown on the right side of the following image.

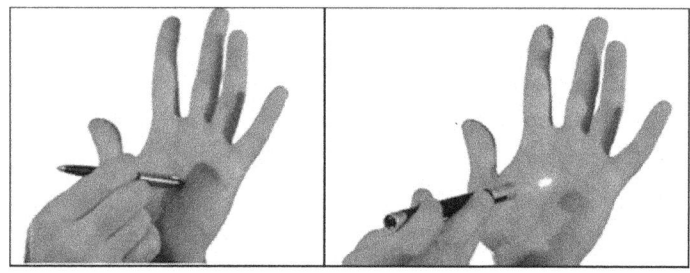

__Different Methods of Acupressure Stimulation:__ The image on the left shows the use of a ball point pen button for acupressure – simply "bounce" the spring-loaded button on the point to be treated.

The image on the right shows laser stimulation. You may simply shine the laser on the point to be treated as shown, or you may touch the pointer directly to the skin.

Regardless of the stimulation method, usually 2 to 3 minutes of stimulation per point is adequate to get results. Longer periods of stimulation are safe, and you can repeat the treatments as often as needed.

Don't let the location of the points confuse you - acupressure points may be nowhere near the site of pain, but they can still be very effective. Some points are used for more than one site of pain. If you aren't sure if you're on the right spot, feel around in the general area where the point should be and you will often find a tender spot that indicates you're on the point. Even if there is no tenderness, you can still benefit from stimulating in the area as close as you can get to the point by following the information in the illustrations that follow.

It is usually most effective to treat the points on the side of the body where the pain is, so if you only have pain on one side, start with the points on that side, but it may be helpful to do the recommended points on both sides of the body, even if the symptoms are only on one side.

Cervical Spinal Stenosis Acupressure Points

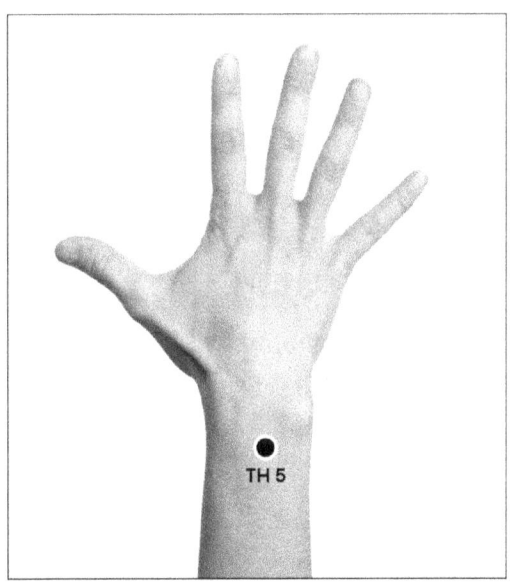

Acupressure Point TH5: Located in the depression between the radius and ulna bones of the forearm (on both arms), two finger widths from the crease at the base of the wrist (bend your wrist backwards to find the crease more easily).

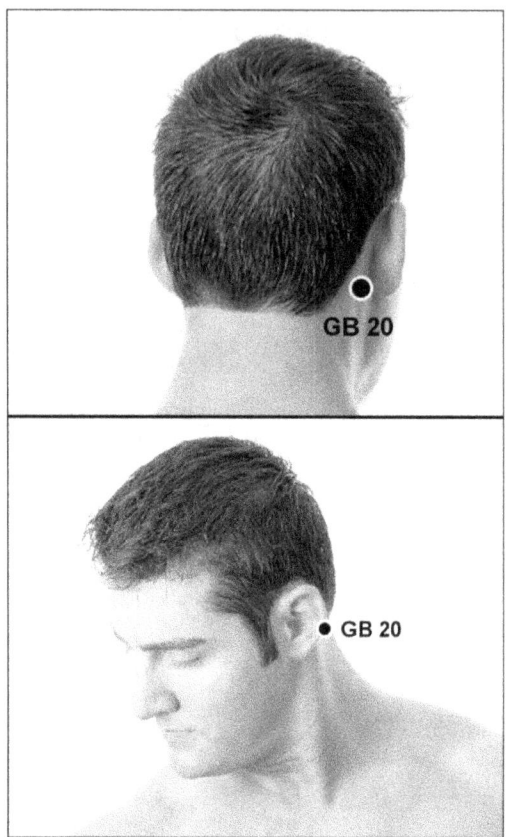

Acupressure Point GB20: *Found at the base of the skull in a depression between the upper portion of the sternocleidomastoid muscle (SCM) and the trapezius muscle, just behind the ear on both sides of the upper neck.*

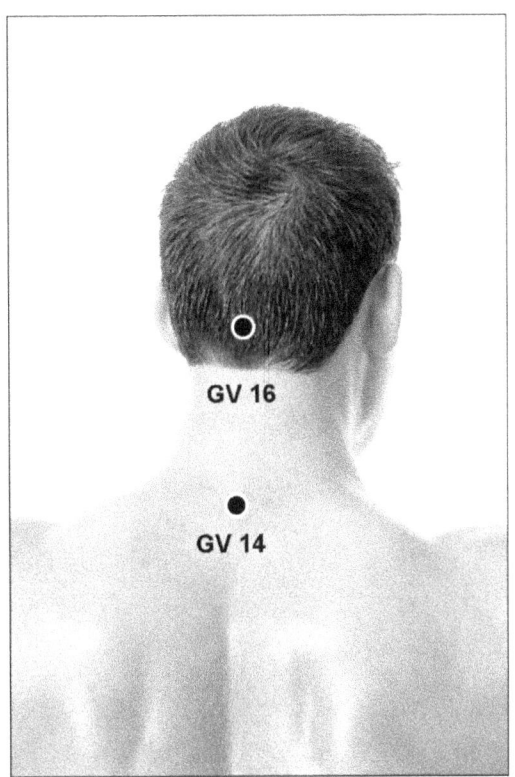

Acupressure Point GV16: *Found in the center of the base of the skull, just below the bony bump at the back of the head known as the external occipital protuberance.*

Acupressure Point GV14: *Located in the middle of the base of the neck on the spinous process of the C7 vertebra. This will usually be the most prominent bony bump at the base of the neck (called the vertebra prominens), but there are cases in which the most prominent bump is either C6 or T1. C7 will be the last vertebra that has a lot of movement when you bend your head forward and backward, and you can use your fingers to feel for it. When in doubt, just stimulate the biggest bony bump, as well as the one above and below it to make sure you get C7.*

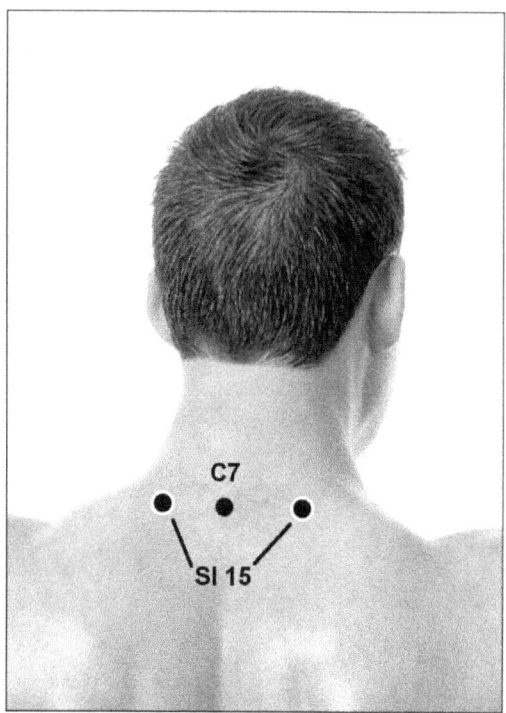

Acupressure Point SI15: *Found on both sides of the spine two finger widths from the C7 spinous process (see acupressure point GV14 in the illustration above for more details on finding the C7 spinous process).*

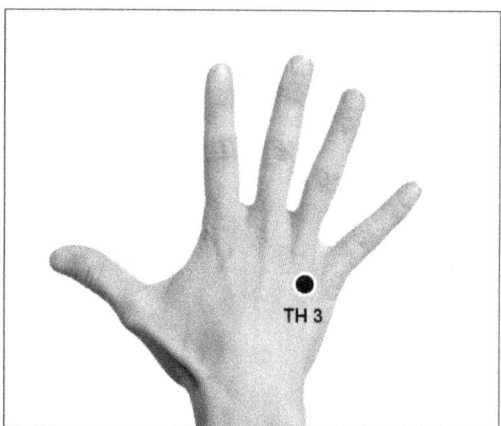

Acupressure point TH3: *Located on the back of each hand just below the knuckle in the depression between the 4th and 5th metacarpal bones (that are in line with the ring and pinky fingers).*

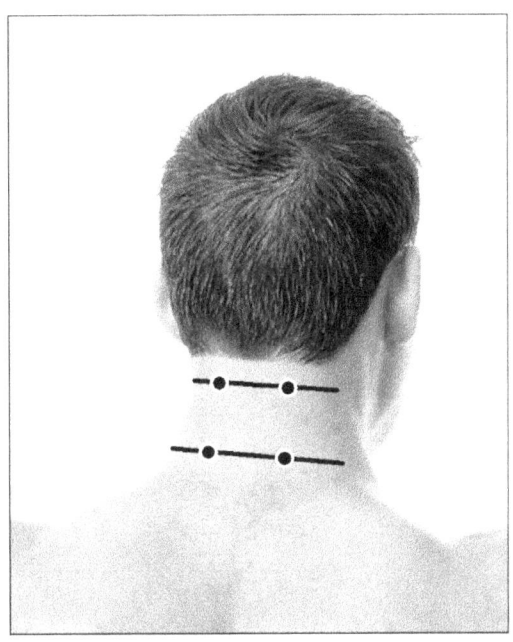

The "Huatuojiaji" Acupressure Points: *Four points that mark the upper and lower boundaries of symptoms in the neck. Using firm fingertip pressure, feel around the neck for tender spots. If any tender points are found, determine the highest and lowest points and imagine a line running across the neck at those points. The four Huatuojiaji points are located at the top (upper Huatuojiaji) and bottom (lower Huatuojiaji) of those lines and one finger width on either side of the spinous process of the cervical vertebra of each line. If only one level of tenderness is identified, select a pair of the Huatuojiaji points on the level of symptoms and a second pair next to the cervical vertebra just below the first pair.*

Lumbar Spinal Stenosis Acupressure Points

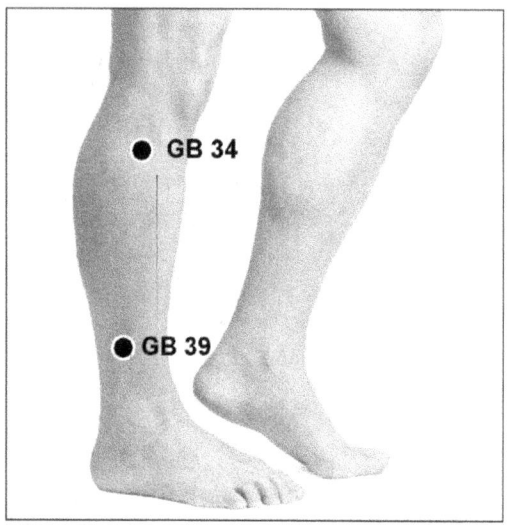

Acupressure Point GB34: *A treatment point that can be used for any type of musculoskeletal pain. It is located about three finger widths below the kneecap on the outside area of the lower leg in a depression just in front of the fibula bone.* ***It is recommended that you begin with this point*** *and then use the other points in whatever order you prefer.*

Acupressure Point GB39*: Located about 3 finger widths above the bone that sticks out on the outside of your ankle at the back edge of the bone. This point is particularly useful when sciatica is present.*

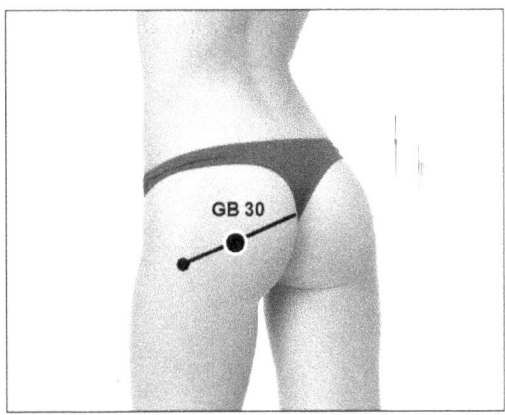

Acupressure Point GB30: *Located in the buttock midway between the hip joint and the tailbone. It is a good point for sciatica.*

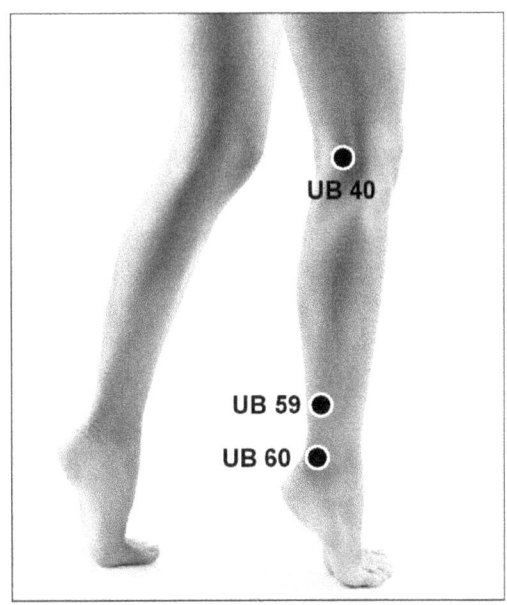

The points above are all useful for relieving spinal stenosis symptoms, particularly low back pain.

Acupressure Point UB40: *Located in the center of the back of the knee at the very lower end of the thigh bone.*

Acupressure Point UB59: *Located just to the outside of the Achilles tendon where it attaches to the lower calf muscle.*

Acupressure Point UB60: *Located just to the outside of the Achilles tendon about 1 finger width above the heel bone.*

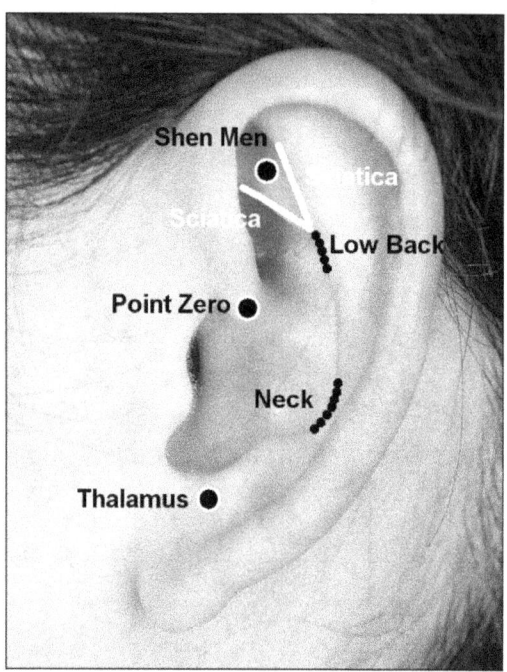

Auriculotherapy (Ear Acupressure) Points: *Shen men, point zero, and the thalamus point can be used for any pain, and the specific areas for the low back, neck, and sciatica are shown. Stimulation of these points is usually accomplished best by either the ball point pen button or laser pointer methods and obviously require a mirror or assistant to see the points.*

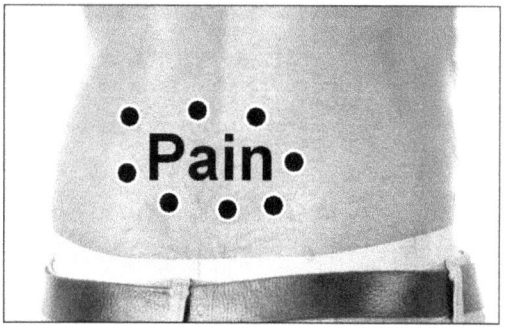

"Surround The Dragon": *This method involves finding tender spots around the site of pain (search the edges of the painful area for points that are tender to touch), and then stimulating them (using any of the methods mentioned previously).*

Chapter 9: Magnets

WARNING

Do not use magnetic therapy products if you have a pacemaker or any other type of electronic implant, as magnets can affect the operation of such devices. Also, as a precaution, avoid magnetic products if you are pregnant (safety in pregnancy is unknown).

Magnetic therapy is somewhat controversial, but there is some research showing benefits from it, and many people find it to be quite helpful for pain relief. Magnetic products range from shoe inserts with magnets built-in (available in both generic and some brands of customized orthotics, such as Foot Levelers which will be discussed in the next chapter), to massage devices, to cards and pads for localized placement, to mattresses and mattress pads.

For the purposes of spinal stenosis, the most useful products are probably shoe inserts, and products designed for localized treatment (small magnetic pads/cards and massagers). There it no one best approach for using magnets. A magnetic pad strapped or taped over the area of stenosis or periodic massage with a magnetic roller or electric massager will often provide good temporary symptom relief. For individuals with a lot of symptoms in their feet and legs, magnetic shoe inserts may work well. For the purposes of trying magnets to see if they help, an inexpensive option is to get a generic pair of magnetic shoe inserts. These can not only be tried in the shoes, but also can be strapped or taped to the area of stenosis to see what effects they have, if any.

Magnetic therapy products range tremendously in cost for what are often very similar products. At the higher end of the price range are Nikken products which are sold through independent distributors in a network marketing business model. Nikken products are excellent quality, but in this author's opinion, they are somewhat expensive compared to other products that are available. An excellent resource for low-cost but still good-quality magnetic products is Lhasa OMS (their website is lhasaoms.com).

One thing that is often overlooked by proponents of magnetic therapy is the potential for overstimulation. In many cases, what happens is initially the magnetic therapy seems to be helping, but after a while of continued use the symptoms not only return, but may even worsen. This simply means that the magnetic therapy has been used too much and it is easily remedied by simply discontinuing the use of the magnet for a little while. As the overstimulation condition eases, the symptoms will once again diminish and then begin to return. At that point, the magnets can be re-applied. With a few cycles, a pattern will usually emerge as to how long the magnets can be used continually without causing a return of symptoms and the overstimulation can be avoided.

Chapter 10: Orthotics

Orthotics (shoe inserts) are often helpful for people with spinal stenosis, particularly when it is in the lumbar region. In many cases, fallen or unstable arches in the feet result in altered skeletal alignment and biomechanics, often increasing mechanical stress on the joints of the low back and pelvis. Good quality orthotics not only support the arches and improve alignment, but also provide some degree of shock-absorption to reduce impact on the discs and joints of the low back.

There are several types of orthotics, ranging from off the shelf arch supports, to semi-customized inserts (such as the Dr. Scholl's "Custom-Fit" orthotics), to fully-customized ones made from detailed scans or casts of the feet.

For many people, general purpose arch supports will actually do a reasonably good job of maintaining skeletal alignment and reducing the symptoms of spinal stenosis. They don't provide a lot of shock-absorption, but given their relatively low cost, they are a good option to try for those on a tight budget.

The next step-up (so to speak) is the semi-custom orthotics. The most widely-available of these are the Dr. Scholl's Custom-Fit orthotics. Kiosks with a foot-mapping device provide a basic analysis of your feet and recommend a specific version of orthotics that are best-suited to your issues. Initially, these had rave reviews, but more recently I've heard complaints that the quality of the product has been significantly downgraded. Given that a set of these inserts typically costs $50 to $60, and may not last more than a few months, they probably are not a good long-term solution, but they can give an indication of whether going to a high-quality fully-customized orthotic is a good investment for you.

Fully-customized orthotics are made on the basis of some type of electronic scan or cast made of your feet. There are various types of these, ranging from a rigid hard plastic variety that is really more for specific foot problems than general musculoskeletal support, to semi-flexible versions that usually have not only good arch support, but excellent shock-absorption as well.

Probably the best-known of the customized orthotics companies is Good Feet. The Good Feet stores employ sales personnel (they are usually not licensed health care practitioners) who will take a history and do an analysis of your feet to make customized recommendations for you. The Good Feet orthotics are generally of good quality, but there have been consumer complaints of "bait and switch" (using a low-cost offer to get you in the store and then selling a much costlier option) and high-pressure sales tactics. In addition, Good Feet uses a three-phase approach to orthotics and depending on your situation, they may recommend up to three different orthotics for you to purchase. This can add up to over $1000, which may very well be worth the cost for some individuals, but in the author's opinion is probably unnecessarily costly in most cases.

One of the more popular brands of semi-flexible orthotics provided by health care professionals is Foot Levelers, which are widely-available through chiropractors and other musculoskeletal specialists. Foot Levelers come in several varieties intended for different activities and types of shoes (for example, they have thinner varieties to fit in dress shoes and thicker, more shock-absorbing ones for athletic shoes). They also make several styles of shoes and sandals with the orthotics built-in. Although they recommend different orthotics for different shoe styles and activities, many of their orthotics are multi-purpose and most people do just fine with a single pair that they simply move from shoe to shoe. The author personally has a single pair of Foot Levelers that he wears in dress oxfords, athletic shoes, and hiking boots and they are still in good shape after several years of daily use (even after getting them soaking wet a few times).

All fully-customized orthotics are relatively expensive (a few hundred dollars and up per pair), but in an overall value sense, a good pair of custom orthotics that lasts at least a few years is a better long-term investment than continual purchases of off the shelf arch supports or semi-custom orthotics that don't hold up nearly as well.

Chapter 11: "Energy Medicine" Techniques

Hopefully you'll forgive the author for going into an area that can seem a bit "weird", but certain "energy medicine" techniques can be nearly miraculous in their effects – when they work. The author was initially hesitant about including them in this book because despite the potential benefits of these techniques, they can seem quite "hokey" to the uninitiated and it's possible that they may call into question the author's credibility with some readers. Even so, since there's little harm in trying them (other than perhaps you may feel a bit silly while doing them) and potentially a big benefit, they have been included in the sections that follow. In the author's 20 plus years of clinical practice, he has seen numerous cases respond to these techniques when all other treatments have failed, so while they may seem a bit odd, the reader is encouraged to give them a try.

As with acupuncture/acupressure, there are various other ways to alter the flow of energy in the body. The first technique that will be presented focuses more on physical energy balance issues responsible for pain, while the second deals more with emotional issues that alter energy flow, but it is recommended that you not make any advance assumptions as to which is more appropriate for your circumstances. It is not unusual for unconscious emotional factors you're completely unaware of to trigger physical pain, so don't be too quick to rule those out even if you're the happiest, most well-adjusted person you know.

Energy Medicine For Physical Pain Relief

This energy medicine technique is a very simplified version of a method the author has used for many years in his chiropractic practice known as Body Restoration Technique (BRT for short). The clinical version of the technique is quite involved in terms of analysis, but in the author's experience, the vast majority of chronic pain cases tend to have the particular pattern about to be presented as a major contributing factor. You will need someone to assist you in doing the procedure and that person's job will be to tap on your back as shown in the directions that follow:

*Note – There are video instructions for this procedure that are more in-depth than the instructions that follow here in the book available at:

www.AskDrBest.com/spinal-stenosis-book-resources

To start the procedure, your assistant positions his/her hand (either hand may be used) as shown so that the fingers and thumb are approximately one inch on either side of the midline of your spine.

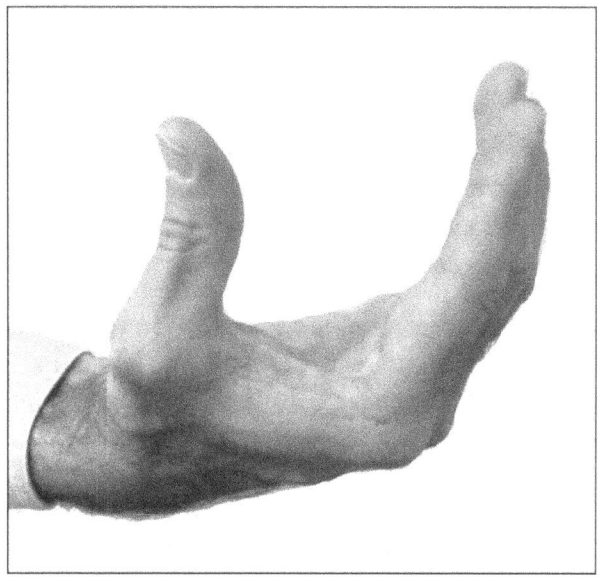

Assistant's Hand Positioning For Tapping Along The Spine

While your assistant taps according the instructions that follow, you will be holding one hand on the area of pain, and a finger from your other hand on your belly button as shown below. Why the belly button? Don't ask, because if you get too caught up in the weirdness of this technique, you probably won't do it and you might miss out on something that could help more than anything else you could do!

Place one of your hands on the area of pain and one finger from your other hand on your belly button. In the case of spinal stenosis, if most of your pain is radiating into your arm or leg, you will usually do best to hold the area of your spinal stenosis (if you know what it is), that is, your neck or low back, rather than the area of pain in the arm or leg, but there is no harm in trying the area of radiating pain on subsequent run-throughs of the technique. Whatever points you are holding, you will hold these points continually as your assistant does the tapping procedure that follows.

While you hold a deep breath, your assistant should begin at the top of your back and rapidly tap with light to moderate pressure (it shouldn't be so hard as to be painful to you) down the spine to your low back, moving down about half an inch with each tap.

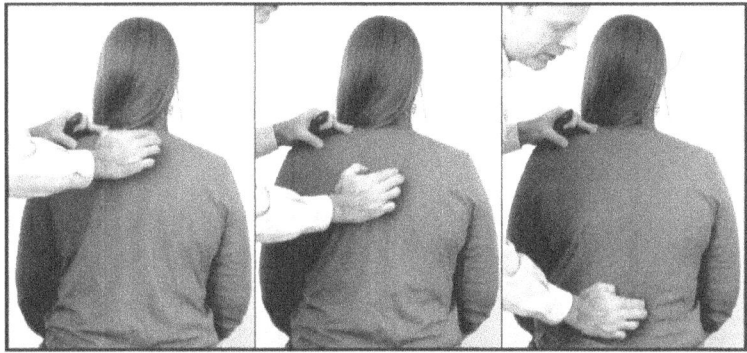

Tapping Procedure: *Your assistant should start at the top of the upper back and tap with light to moderate pressure at approximately ½ inch intervals down your spine to the lower back.*

Next, as you breathe out, your assistant starts again at the top of your back and taps down the spine to your low back. Finally, as you breathe in and out rapidly (in and out about once every second), your assistant taps once more down the spine as before.

After going through the first round of holding the points and getting tapped on, re-assess the area of pain. In many cases, the location of pain will change somewhat. If so, re-position your hand to cover the new area of pain, or move it up or down on your neck or back if you know the general area your stenosis is in. If it requires some pressure to produce tenderness, go ahead and press on it just hard enough to produce a bit of pain, make sure to hold your belly button with your other hand, and then have your assistant repeat the procedure of tapping with the three breathing phases.

Each time through, re-assess the pain area, relocate your hand to hold any new areas of pain as before (or move up or down on the area you know your stenosis is located in), and repeat the process. Continue repeating until you either no longer have any pain, or until you stop getting any improvement.

If you don't ever get any improvement with this method after 3 or 4 tries, it's probably not going to work for you, so there's not much point in continuing. In a few cases, there is a delayed response of up to 2 days though, so if your symptoms suddenly improve in that time frame and then gradually return for no apparent reason, it may be worth trying this method again.

Be aware that after an initial relief of pain, the pain may return and even possibly get worse sometime in the next 1 to 2 days. If so, repeat the process and try the fine-tuning procedures shown on the video available at:

http://www.AskDrBest.com/spinal-stenosis-book-resources

It may take several sessions to get permanent relief of the symptoms, but as long as each session provides temporary relief, it is worthwhile to continue.

Energy Medicine for Emotional Stress Management (EFT):

It is not uncommon for physical pain and other symptoms to be triggered or increased by emotional factors, so the better you can manage your emotional stress, the better you'll likely be able to manage your physical symptoms as well. There are many methods for handling negative emotional states. Some people do well with meditation, positive affirmations, and other "mental" approaches, while others do better using physical activity to dissipate stress. One simple method that somewhat combines the mental and physical aspects of stress-management and that is well-suited to self-treatment is called Emotional Freedom Technique, or EFT for short.

Emotional Freedom Technique is most often used as a means of handling negative emotions and as a means of habit control, but it can be very helpful in dealing with pain as well. EFT combines acupressure with verbal affirmations to change your emotional state. The basic procedure is summarized here and most people will do quite well just using the basics, but you can also download a free full-length manual on this method, as well as get information on seminars and advanced instruction by going to www.EFTuniverse.com.

As was just mentioned, Emotional Freedom Technique uses acupressure stimulation along with verbal affirmations to change the "emotional charge" or intensity of a physical pain, craving, habit, phobia, or traumatic event. The starting point of the procedure is to identify whatever it is you want to change, and then verbalize it in the form of a self-accepting affirmation while tapping a series of points.

For example, let's say you are experiencing sciatica. For the purposes of doing Emotional Freedom Technique, you will always use the structure of "Even though I [insert undesirable symptom, behavior, or emotion here], I deeply and completely accept myself." So, using the example of sciatica, you would say, "Even though I am having sciatica, I deeply and completely accept myself."

In the case of pain and other symptoms, you may be able to associate a certain emotional event or stressful situation to the onset or increase of the symptoms. In fact, sometimes simply noticing the words we use can clue us in on emotional issues that may be triggering physical symptoms.

Even though most symptoms of spinal stenosis are related to objective physical abnormalities in the spine, you might be surprised at how much of a role emotional issues can play. For instance, if you are unhappy at work and think your boss is a "pain in the butt", you may very well experience increased physical sciatica pain in the buttock area when you have to deal with your boss.

Diminishing the "charge" of underlying emotional issues can bring a surprising amount of pain relief in some cases. Although other techniques for using affirmations may recommend phrasing your affirmations in terms of the way you want things to be (such as, "I feel healthy and pain-free!"), this is not how they are used with Emotional Freedom Technique. So, as another example, let's say that you recognize that emotional issues from dealing with your boss may be participating in your physical symptoms, you could use the affirmation, "Even though I feel like my boss is a pain in the butt, I deeply and completely accept myself."

Whatever the affirmation for your specific issue, you repeat it out loud as you tap a series of acupressure points. The sequence and location of the points is shown on the next page. For each point, you'll tap it 7 or 8 times with a finger tip as you repeat the affirmation out loud. Tap the points in the number sequence shown, starting at point 1 above the eye and working through to point 13 (if you download the full manual from the Emotional Freedom Technique website, you'll see that I have added one finger point – this point is optional and I have included it only because it is easier to just do all of the fingers than try to remember which one you don't need to do).

It usually does not matter whether you do points on the left or right side of the body, but I find it usually works better to stick to one side, rather than doing some points on the left and some on the right. You may find that tapping the points on the side of pain works the best.

Points For Emotional Freedom Technique

(The points are illustrated above, indicated as dots on the pictures.)

1. Over Eye

2. Outside Corner Of Eye

3. Under Eye

4. Between Nose And Upper Lip

5. Between Lower Lip And Chin

6. Just Below Where Collar Bone Joins Breastbone

7. Center Of Arm Pit

8. Outer Edge Of Base Of Thumb Nail

9. Outer Edge (Thumb Side) Of Base Of Index Finger Nail

10. Outer Edge (Thumb Side) Of Base Of Middle Finger Nail

11. Outer Edge (Thumb Side) Of Base Of Ring Finger Nail

12. Outer Edge (Thumb Side) Of Base Of Little ("Pinky") Finger Nail

13. "Karate Chop" Point On Outer Edge Of Hand Midway Between Little Finger and Wrist

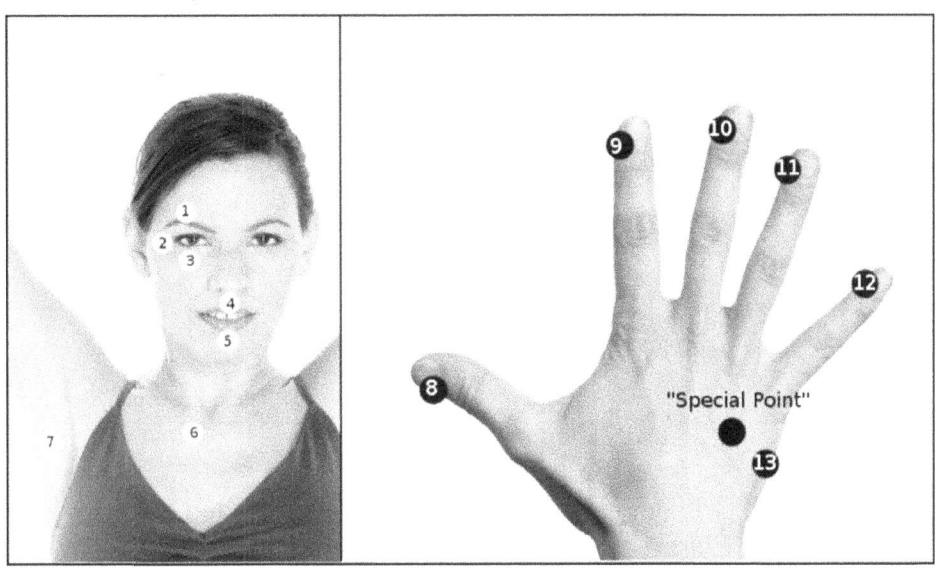

Points For Emotional Freedom Technique:

1. Over Eye

2. Outside Corner Of Eye

3. Under Eye

4. Between Nose And Upper Lip

5. Between Lower Lip And Chin

6. Just Below Where Collar Bone Joins Breastbone

7. Center Of Arm Pit

8. Outer Edge Of Base Of Thumb Nail

9. Outer Edge (Thumb Side) Of Base Of Index Finger Nail

10. Outer Edge (Thumb Side) Of Base Of Middle Finger Nail

11. Outer Edge (Thumb Side) Of Base Of Ring Finger Nail

12. Outer Edge (Thumb Side) Of Base Of Little ("Pinky") Finger Nail

13. "Karate Chop" Point On Outer Edge Of Hand Midway Between Little Finger and Wrist

"Special Point" – See Instructions That Follow.

After you have tapped on the series of points while repeating the affirmation ("Even though I [insert undesirable symptom, behavior, or emotion here], I deeply and completely accept myself."), the next step is to activate various brain centers while tapping on what I'll call the "special point" point on the back of the hand, on a line directly between the ring finger and little finger, midway between the base of the fingers and the wrist (as shown on the hand image in the previous picture).

As you tap on the "special point", you'll go through a series of steps as follows:

1. Open your eyes.

2. Close your eyes.

3. Open your eyes and, without moving your head, look down and left with your eyes.

4. Open your eyes and, without moving your head, look down and right with your eyes.

5. Circle ("roll") your eyes clockwise.

6. Circle ("roll") your eyes counter-clockwise.

7. Hum a tune for a few seconds (any familiar tune will work, such as the "Happy Birthday" song).

8. Count out loud from one to five ("one, two, three, four, five").

9. Hum a tune again for a few seconds.

Once you have completed these procedures while tapping the "special point", there's one more step. Once again, you will tap 7 or 8 times on each of the 13 points done in the initial step, this time while repeating just the phrase that describes the undesirable symptom, habit, behavior, or emotion. For example, if your affirmation in the first step of the procedure was, "Even though I have sciatica, I deeply and completely accept myself," this time through you will repeat just the phrase, "sciatica" while you tap the points.

After one time through the entire procedure, most people will have significant improvement in the symptoms, habit, behavior, or emotion they wish to change. If there is no improvement, you may want to think about underlying issues that are related to the problem you wish to address. For example, if your pain started shortly after a major fight with your wife about your finances, you might switch from a symptom-focused affirmation like "Even though I have sciatica…" to "Even though I disagree with my wife about our finances…".

If there is some, but not 100% improvement, the procedure can be repeated with a variation in the affirmation used in the initial step and the phrase used in the final step. For repeats of the procedure, there is an acknowledgment of the prior issue being somewhat improved.

For example, if the first time through the procedure your affirmation was, "Even though I have sciatica, I deeply and completely accept myself.", your affirmation for the first step each time you repeat the procedure will be, "Even though I **still** have **some remaining** sciatica, I deeply and completely accept myself.". And for the final step of the procedure for the repeats, the phrase would change from "sciatica" to "**remaining** sciatica". Otherwise, the procedure for repeats is the same as when you do it the first time for a given issue.

In some cases, you may need to get more specific with your affirmation to help with the problem you are experiencing. For instance, if you are having problems with left buttock pain, it may be more effective to say, "Even though I have pain in my left buttock…" than to say "Even though I have sciatica…". The more specific you can be and the more you can deal with any possible emotional triggers for your pain, the more effective EFT will be.

Chapter 12: Exercises

The most effective exercises for reducing spinal stenosis symptoms are often more positions than exercises in the traditional sense. In the author's experience, most people who attempt to use exercises to alleviate symptoms fail to do them frequently enough to get maximum benefit. Even recommendations from doctors and physical therapists usually are inadequate to get the desired results as quickly as may be possible with a more intensive regimen.

Because of this generally low-intensity approach to exercises that may be familiar, the exercise recommendations that follow may seem a bit extreme in terms of frequency. Bear in mind that the exercises are intended not only to improve symptoms but, when possible, to actually bring about physical improvements in the underlying causes of your stenosis. Achieving that type of lasting change in the involved tissues requires an intensive approach initially. As your condition improves, the frequency of the exercise can be decreased until you reach a prevention stage which only requires a few minutes per day to maintain.

Exercises For Cervical Spine Stenosis:

The first thing to take into consideration is whether the problem is central canal or intervertebral stenosis. As stated previously, it is recommended that you do not perform any of the exercises that follow if you have been diagnosed with severe cervical central canal stenosis (you may try the methods that follow with mild to moderate central canal stenosis).

The McKenzie Method for the Cervical Spine

Again, if you have been diagnosed with SEVERE central canal stenosis, you should NOT attempt any of the self-treatment methods that follow without your doctor's approval. These methods are intended for intervertebral stenosis and mild to moderate cases of central stenosis only!

It is recommended that you go through the full testing procedure for the McKenzie Method that follows; however, the starting point for testing may vary depending on the site and cause of your stenosis. The testing procedure has been simplified somewhat from what would be done by a professional trained in the McKenzie Method to make it easier to use for self-assessment. If you get some, but not complete improvement using the McKenzie Method, it may be worthwhile to seek out the help of a physician or physical therapist certified in its use.

Stenosis (central or intervertebral) caused primarily by posterior element conditions (bone spurring/thickening and/or ligament thickening/buckling) will usually respond best to protrusion or flexion, so those positions should be tested first in those circumstances.

On the other hand, central and/or intervertebral stenosis caused primarily by a disc protrusion will usually respond best to one of the retraction or extension positions, so I recommend you test those first if you know that a disc protrusion is a significant factor in your case. If one of those positions does prove effective, there is no need to test the protrusion and flexion positions.

The lateral flexion and rotation positions should be tested in any case, but it is recommended that these be done after protrusion/flexion (for posterior element stenosis) or retraction/extension (for disc-related stenosis). Although lateral flexion and/or rotation may be helpful and important, they may provide more of a "fine-tuning" of improvement as compared to more dramatic results from the movements in the front to back planes.

In cases where both disc and posterior element factors are producing the stenosis, it may be necessary to alternate the protraction/flexion and retraction/extension positions periodically. In this situation, test all positions and begin by using whichever worked the best. If at some point that position is no longer helpful or actually seems to increase symptoms, re-test (all of the positions) and change to the new best position(s) you find. This process of switching positions will likely continue for some time if you are having stenosis from both the front and back portions of the effected spinal canal(s).

In cases of mild to moderate central stenosis due primarily to bone thickening, the McKenzie exercises may not be effective long-term, as in such cases the involved structures are not as readily changeable as with disc and ligament related stenosis. The McKenzie positions are still worth testing as they do help in some cases of bony stenosis (primarily providing short-term relief), but if you are not finding any position that seems beneficial, simply focus on the other self-treatment methods in this book initially and perhaps try the McKenzie method again when things are feeling better.

Centralization

There is a very important concept you need to be familiar with in regards to using the McKenzie method known as *centralization*. Centralization means that the symptoms furthest from the spine improve, even if other symptoms closer to the spine worsen at the same time. When testing the McKenzie positions, initially you are looking for the **one** position that **best centralizes** the symptoms.

For example, if you have pain extending down your arm all the way to your wrist, you are looking for the position that best reduces the pain in your wrist (and then produces gradual improvements moving up the arm), even if that position initially makes your neck or upper arm feel worse.

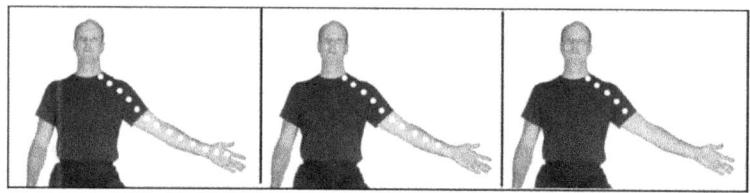

Centralization of Arm Symptoms

If you have symptoms going down your leg to your ankle, you are looking for the position that reduces the ankle pain first, and then reduces the pain in the lower leg, the thigh, then the buttocks.

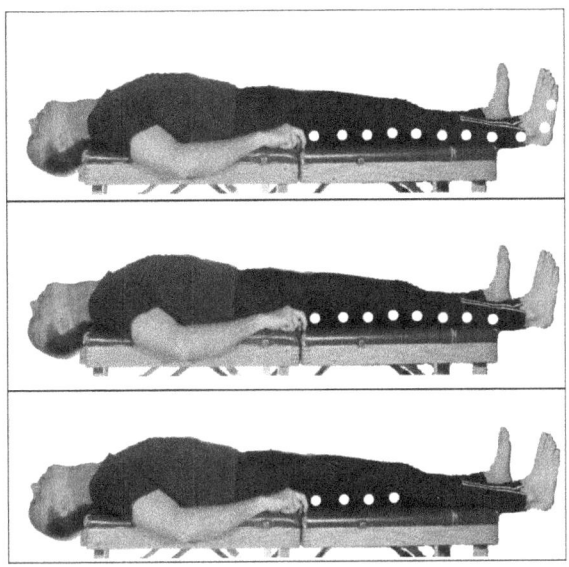

Centralization of Leg Symptoms

Of course, if your symptoms are localized and don't extend out from the spine much or at all, you are then looking for the position that best reduces your symptoms.

The opposite of centralization is peripheralization, meaning the symptoms furthest from the spine increase and/or the symptoms extend further from the spine than initially. Just keep in mind, centralization is good and a sign to continue with what you are doing and perpheralization is bad and a sign to stop.

As a reminder of the previous discussion of the relative severity of pain and numbness, generally speaking, numbness is worse than pain (in terms of neurological function). So, a transition from numbness to pain (or tingling, burning, or other sensation) in the area of symptoms furthest from the spine is still centralization and is a positive sign.

As you continue to perform the exercise/position, the symptoms should gradually improve from furthest from the spine to closest to the spine and hopefully go away altogether. Lasting elimination of symptoms can take anywhere from a few minutes to a few months of performing the exercise, depending on the severity of the underlying problems. For best results when major symptoms are present, it is recommended that the exercise/position be done for short durations on a frequent basis – thirty seconds to a minute at a time up to 5 or 6 times every hour you are awake. That was not a misprint – for best results, provided that centralization is occurring (or localized symptoms are improving), you should try to do the exercise up to **5 or 6 times every hour you are awake** (or as often as possible if you can't do it that much)! You may experience some muscle soreness doing it that much, but as long as the symptoms are centralizing and any localized intense pain is diminishing, you are on the right track. In most cases, this intensive treatment regimen will bring about lasting relief within a few weeks (usually within a few days), at which point you may begin gradually reducing the frequency. Even once symptoms are completely gone, a preventive regimen of a minute or two once or twice a day is strongly recommended to avoid a return of symptoms.

Once again, when testing the positions that follow, you are looking for the ONE position that best centralizes the symptoms. There may be a brief twinge of increased symptoms when you first get into the position, even if it is a good one, so give it a moment to allow things to "settle" before assessing the amount of centralization / symptom improvement. If there is no clear "winner", it is recommended that you start by using the retraction with extension position if you have a disc protrusion, or the straight flexion position if you have more of a posterior element stenosis (as discussed previously in this book).

For each position shown, start by slowly getting into the position, hold it for a few seconds, and then relax / return to the neutral position. As long as there was no peripheralization of the symptoms (increased symptoms furthest from the spine and/or symptoms extending further from the spine) on the first repetition, repeat the movement into the position 10 times or so (holding for a few seconds each time)and note the results. If you find one of the positions/movements that centralizes and improves your symptoms better than all of the others, you may discontinue testing at this point and simply use that movement/position repeatedly as your exercise. Remember, for best results, do the exercise frequently – a few times every hour you are awake, if possible – until the symptoms are mostly to completely gone and then transition to a lowered frequency of doing the exercise to perhaps a few times each day.

Now, if none of the movements/positions produced significant centralization, the next step is to test a bit further to see if you can find a position that does produce centralization. As before, you will position yourself as shown in each of the pictures that follow (skipping any that peripheralized your symptoms – intensified and/or extended them further from the spine - in the first stage of the testing), but this time you will hold the end position for 30 seconds to a minute to see which, if any, of the positions will best-centralize your symptoms. If you find a position that does produce good centralization, you may use it frequently throughout the day (a few times every hour you are awake is optimal in most cases), holding the end position for a minute or so each time.

Remember, if you found one of the movements provided good centralization, you don't need to do the tests of staying in the positions for longer periods of time, and you may proceed directly to using the movement frequently throughout the day. Adding in a few sessions of longer holds of the positon is fine and possibly helpful if you wish to do it in these circumstances, but it is not absolutely necessary for good results.

To summarize, test the movements/positions shown below. When you find a movement/position that centralizes your symptoms (or improves them if they are localized around the spine to begin with), use that movement/position frequently throughout the day (preferably at least once every hour you are awake). Once your symptoms are gone or much-improved for a few days, you can reduce the frequency of doing the movement/position to a few times every day for prevention, and just do the more "intensive" program if you have a return of the symptoms at some point.

The McKenzie Method Cervical Spine Positions

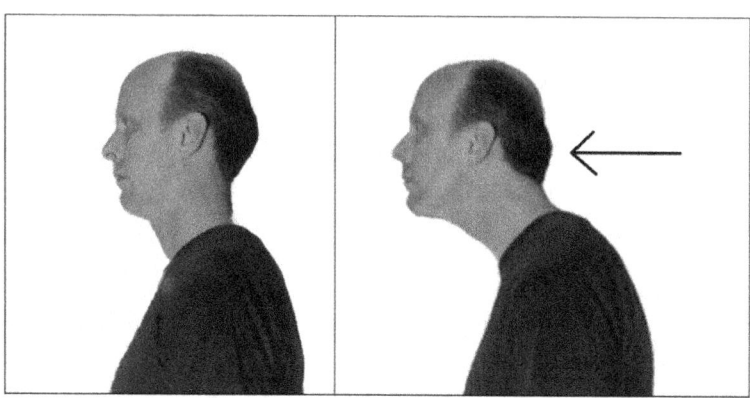

Protrusion: *Start with your head in a comfortable upright position and, keeping your head upright and eyes straight ahead, slide your head straight forward as shown. Hold in this position for a few seconds, and then relax / return to the neutral position. If there was no peripheralization of the symptoms (increased symptoms furthest from the spine and/or symptoms extending further from the spine) on the first repetition, repeat the movement into the position 10 times or so (holding for a few seconds each time) and note the results. If you experience centralization of your symptoms (a decrease in symptoms furthest from the spine or decrease in symptoms overall if you only have localized symptoms) with this position, note the amount of improvement to compare to the other positions you test. Discontinue testing this position if at any time you experience peripheralization of symptoms.*

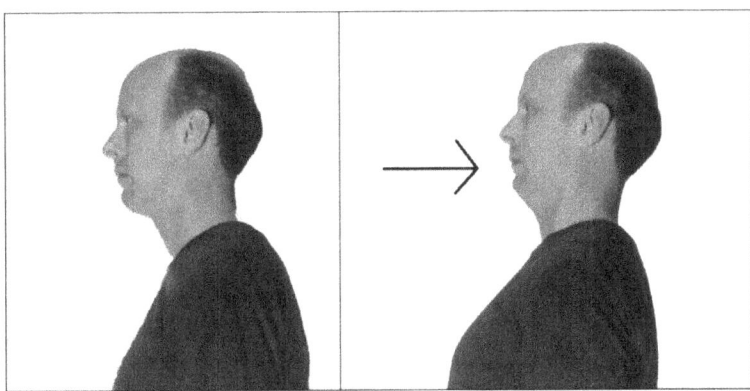

Retraction: _Start with your head in a comfortable upright position and, keeping your head upright and eyes straight ahead, slide your head straight backwards and tucking your chin as shown. Hold in this position for a few seconds, and then relax / return to the neutral position._ _If there was no peripheralization of the symptoms (increased symptoms furthest from the spine and/or symptoms extending further from the spine) on the first repetition, repeat the movement into the position 10 times or so (holding for a few seconds each time) and note the results. If you experience centralization of your symptoms (a decrease in symptoms furthest from the spine or decrease in symptoms overall if you only have localized symptoms) with this position, note the amount of improvement to compare to the other positions you test. Discontinue testing this position if at any time you experience peripheralization of symptoms._

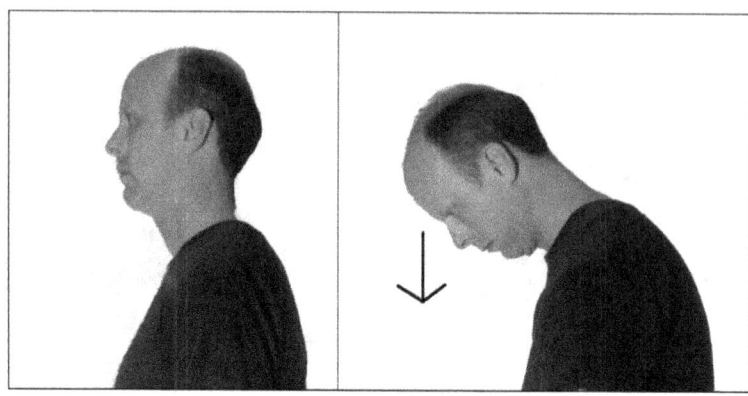

Flexion: Start with your head in a comfortable upright position and slowly bend your head forward and down as shown. Hold in this position for a few seconds, and then relax / return to the neutral position. If there was no peripheralization of the symptoms (increased symptoms furthest from the spine and/or symptoms extending further from the spine) on the first repetition, repeat the movement into the position 10 times or so (holding for a few seconds each time) and note the results. If you experience centralization of your symptoms (a decrease in symptoms furthest from the spine or decrease in symptoms overall if you only have localized symptoms) with this position, note the amount of improvement to compare to the other positions you test. Discontinue testing this position if at any time you experience peripheralization of symptoms.

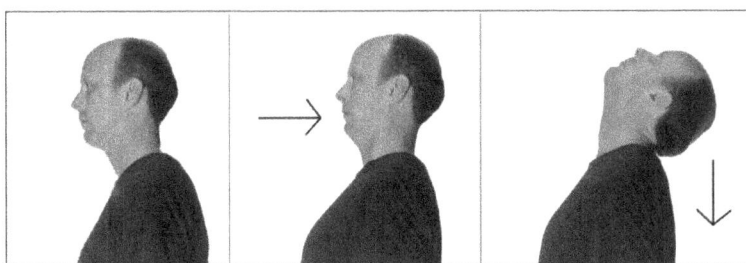

Retraction With Extension (Sitting): *Start with your head in a comfortable upright position and, keeping your head upright and eyes straight ahead, first slide your head straight backward as shown, then at the end of that movement, tip your head back and down as shown. Hold in this position for a few seconds, and then relax / return to the neutral position. If there was no peripheralization of the symptoms (increased symptoms furthest from the spine and/or symptoms extending further from the spine) on the first repetition, repeat the movement into the position 10 times or so (holding for a few seconds each time) and note the results. If you experience centralization of your symptoms (a decrease in symptoms furthest from the spine or decrease in symptoms overall if you only have localized symptoms) with this position, note the amount of improvement to compare to the other positions you test. Discontinue testing this position if at any time you experience peripheralization of symptoms.*

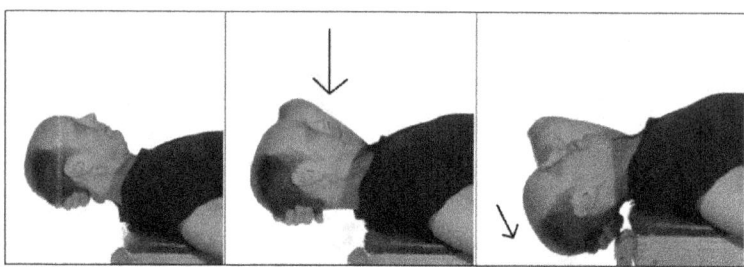

Retraction With Extension (Lying Down): *Start by lying on your back with your head supported in a comfortable position. The support can be done using your own hand as shown, or you can have someone else assist you with this. Having an assistant is recommended if you have difficulty getting in and out of the lying down position.*

From the starting position, keep your chin tucked and gently press your head straight backwards as shown and from the end point of this movement continue by tipping your head backwards. Hold in this position for a few seconds, and then relax / return to the neutral position. If there was no peripheralization of the symptoms (increased symptoms furthest from the spine and/or symptoms extending further from the spine) on the first repetition, repeat the movement into the position 10 times or so (holding for a few seconds each time) and note the results. If you experience centralization of your symptoms (a decrease in symptoms furthest from the spine or decrease in symptoms overall if you only have localized symptoms) with this position, note the amount of improvement to compare to the other positions you test. Discontinue testing this position if at any time you experience peripheralization of symptoms.

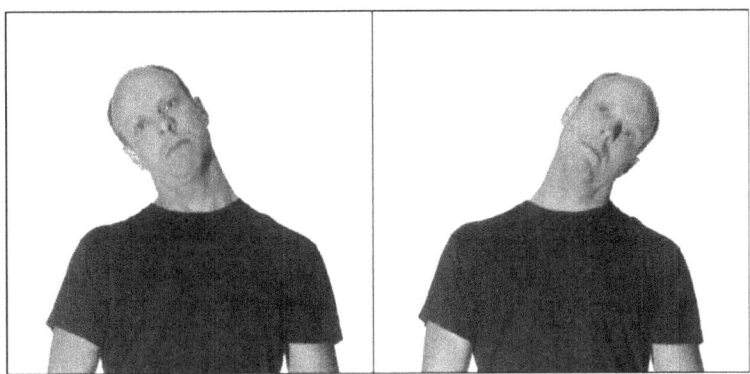

Lateral Flexion: *Start with your head in a comfortable upright position and then bend it to one side as shown. Hold in this position for a few seconds, and then relax / return to the neutral position.   If there was no peripheralization of the symptoms (increased symptoms furthest from the spine and/or symptoms extending further from the spine) on the first repetition, repeat the movement into the same position (bending to the same side) 10 times or so (holding for a few seconds each time) and note the results. If you experience centralization of your symptoms (a decrease in symptoms furthest from the spine or decrease in symptoms overall if you only have localized symptoms) with this position, note the amount of improvement to compare to the other positions you test. Discontinue testing this position if at any time you experience peripheralization of symptoms. Repeat the procedure above with bending to the opposite side.*

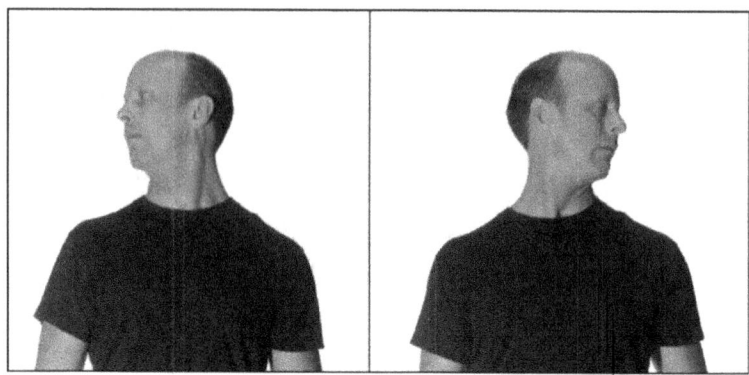

Rotation: *Start with your head in a comfortable upright position and then turn it to one side as shown. Hold in this position for a few seconds, and then relax / return to the neutral position. If there was no peripheralization of the symptoms (increased symptoms furthest from the spine and/or symptoms extending further from the spine) on the first repetition, repeat the movement into the same position (turning to the same side) 10 times or so (holding for a few seconds each time) and note the results. If you experience centralization of your symptoms (a decrease in symptoms furthest from the spine or decrease in symptoms overall if you only have localized symptoms) with this position, note the amount of improvement to compare to the other positions you test. Discontinue testing this position if at any time you experience peripheralization of symptoms. Repeat the procedure above with turning to the opposite side.*

Once you have tested the various positions, try to decide on which position provided the best centralization of your symptoms (decrease in symptoms furthest from the spine) or improvement in symptoms if they were localized close to the spine to begin with. Whichever ONE position BEST centralized/improved the symptoms, that is the position you will use initially to help reduce your symptoms. If none of the positions provided centralization/improvement, you will not use any of the positions and it is recommended that you stick with the other self-treatment methods (cold packs, acupressure, etc.) and your prescribed treatment from your healthcare provider(s).

If you did find a position that did a good job of centralizing/improving your symptoms, it is recommended that you use it frequently at first to get the maximum improvement in your symptoms as quickly as possible. As a starting point, the author suggests doing whichever position/movement best centralized symptoms for 10 repetitions (holding the end position for a few seconds on each repetition) at least two or three times every hour you are awake (and up to five or six times is even better).

While you will usually be sticking with the one position you initially found that best centralized your symptoms, in some cases things change and a position/movement that initially worked well will stop helping or possibly even begin to peripheralize or worsen symptoms. If this occurs, simply go back through the testing procedure and try to find a new position that will once again centralize your symptoms.

Cervical Flexibility and Alignment Exercises

General flexibility and good skeletal alignment can significantly reduce mechanical stresses on the structures of the cervical spine and greatly reduce symptoms of spinal stenosis. In addition, some symptoms attributed to spinal stenosis may actually be coming from trigger points (knots of contraction that cause referred pain) in the muscles of the cervical and upper thoracic regions and the exercises that follow will usually be very helpful for reducing muscular symptoms.

Some of the exercises that follow are identical to positions tested in the McKenzie Method, but the use and purpose is different. These exercises are intended primarily for maintenance and prevention rather than for treating severe symptoms. It is strongly recommended that you work with the McKenzie Method procedures in the previous section first to try to get any major symptoms under control before you begin using the general flexibility and alignment exercises that follow. Once your symptoms have been greatly reduced or eliminated for at least a week, you may try the general flexibility and alignment exercises.

As was just stated, the exercises that follow are intended for maintenance and prevention. It is recommended that you also continue the McKenzie position/movement that best centralized symptomson a preventive basis, in addition to the exercises that follow. Unlike the "intensive care" recommendations for the McKenzie Method when major symptoms are present, when used for maintenance and prevention the recommended frequency is one session of ten repetitions or so once or twice per day, rather than multiple times per hour.

Proceed slowly and gently with the following exercises when you first attempt them and immediately discontinue any that cause peripheralized symptoms (that extend further from the spine or worsen at the point furthest from the spine) or increased symptoms when they start out localized.

The one exception to the peripheralization restriction is the scalene stretch. When stretched, the scalene muscles commonly cause referred symptoms into the arm, shoulder blade, and/or chest (the symptom pattern can mimic the feelings of a heart attack). As long as the lateral flexion and extension stretches did not produce any peripheralization of symptoms, you may proceed with the scalene stretch even if there is an initial peripheralization of symptoms as you begin the stretch. If you do get peripheralization of symptoms as you begin the scalene stretch, the symptoms should begin to centralize and improve after a few repetitions. If they do not, you should then discontinue the stretch (unless advised to do it by your doctor or physical therapist).

Here are the positions for cervical flexibility and alignment:

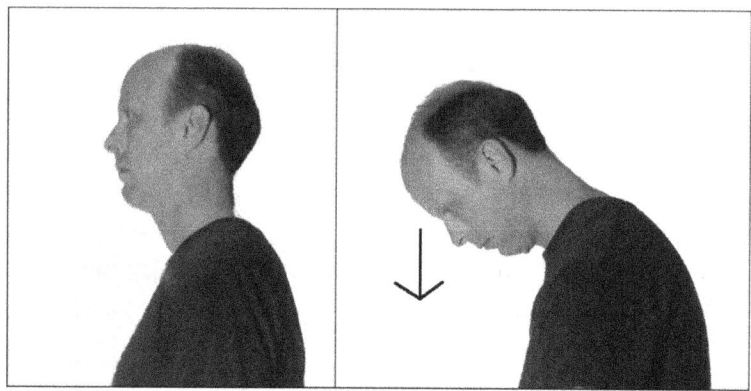

Cervical Flexion: Bend your head forward as far as you can go without pain and hold for 10 to 30 seconds. Return to the starting position and repeat 5 to10 times.

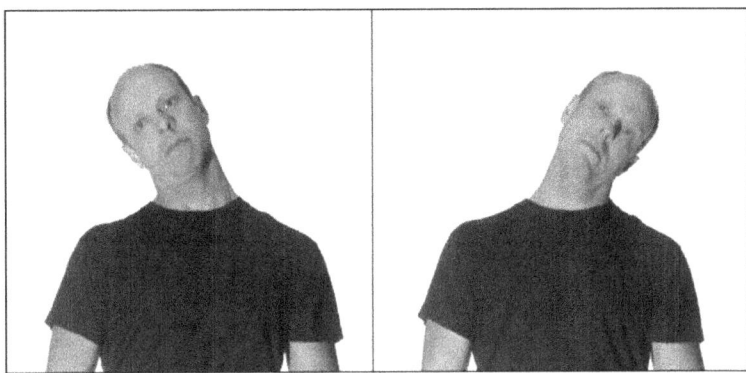

Cervical Lateral Flexion (Side-bending): *Bend your head to one side as far as you can go without pain and hold for 10 to 30 seconds. Return to the starting position and then bend your head to the opposite side and hold for 10 to 30 seconds. Repeat 5 to10 times on each side.*

It's a good idea to do this stretch in front of a mirror and observe the relative range of motion from one side to the other. If there is a significant difference in the range of motion, it may be helpful to increase the number of repetitions on the more restricted side. For example, if you can bend to the right further than you can to the left, it may be helpful to do two repetitions bending to the left for every one you do bending to the right.

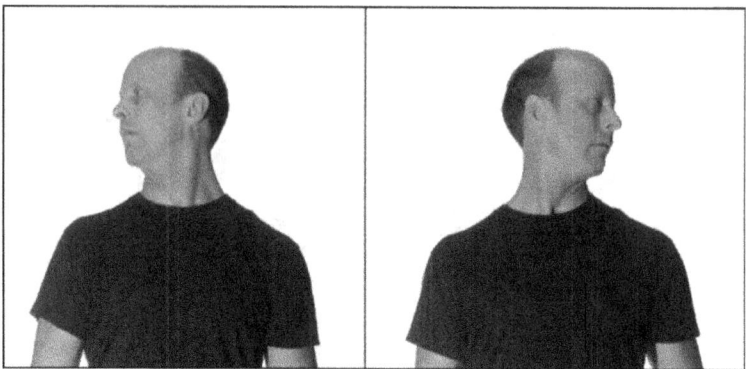

Cervical Rotation: *Turn your head to one side as far as you can go without pain and hold for 10 to 30 seconds. Return to the starting position and then turn your head to the opposite side and hold for 10 to 30 seconds. Repeat 5 to 10 times on each side.*

It's a good idea to do this stretch in front of a mirror (standing facing the mirror as well as with each side to the mirror so that you are facing it at the end of the rotation movement) and observe the relative range of motion from one side to the other. If there is a significant difference in the range of motion, it may be helpful to increase the number of repetitions on the more restricted side. For example, if you can turn to the right further than you can to the left, it may be helpful to do two repetitions turning to the left for every one you do turning to the right.

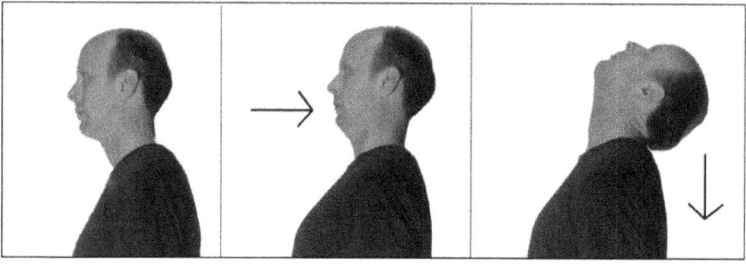

Cervical Extension: *Begin by doing a head retraction, keeping your head level and sliding your head backwards as far as you can go comfortably and then continue the movement by bending your head backwards as far as you can go without pain and hold for 10 to 30 seconds. Return to the starting position and repeat 5 to 10 times.*

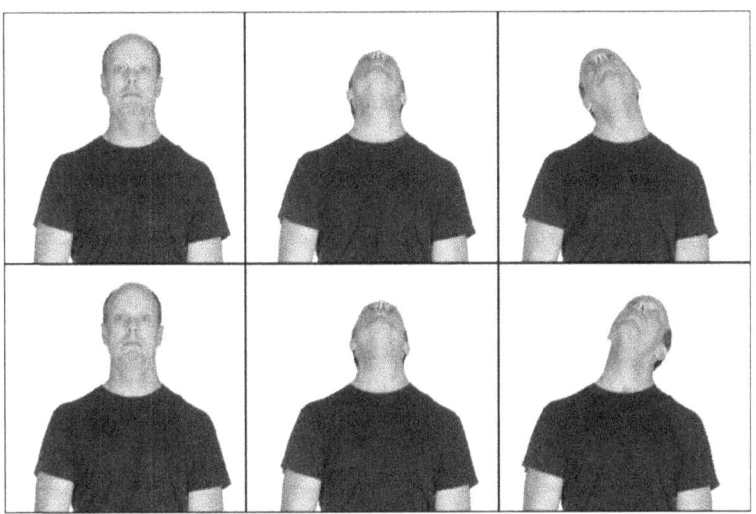

Scalene Stretch: *Do NOT attempt if you have moderate to severe stenosis due to bone spurs!*

Begin by performing the cervical extension as shown in the previous exercise and then continue the motion by bending your head to one side as far as you can go without pain and hold for 10 to 30 seconds. Return to the starting position and repeat the steps with bending to the opposite side.

***Warning:** Discontinue this exercise immediately if you experience any lightheadedness, dizziness, or nausea, as these may be signs of diminished circulation to the brain. If such symptoms occur, it is strongly advised that you seek professional evaluation of the blood vessels in your neck at your earliest opportunity and avoid activities and positons that place your neck in an extended and rotated position.*

Exercises For Lumbar Spine Stenosis:

The McKenzie Method

As we've already discussed with regards to the cervical spine, the key to the McKenzie Method is in finding the one position that best centralizes the symptoms.

Centralization

In the picture below, the concept of centralization is illustrated once again as it relates to the lumbar spine, with the stars representing the extension of symptoms down the leg. In the top image, the initial symptoms extend all the way to the foot, but as symptoms centralize the symptoms leave the foot and lower leg and gradually decrease and work their way up towards the spine - as shown in the bottom image.

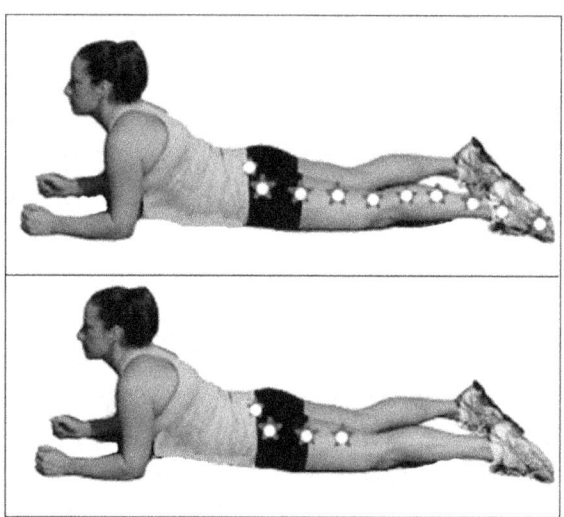

Centralization of Symptoms Associated With Lumbar Stenosis

Over time, in most cases the thigh, buttock, and low back pain will also improve in situations where initial centralization is achieved. As with the cervical spine, the opposite of centralization is peripheralization in which the symptoms furthest from the spine increase and/or extend further from the spine than initially - a bad sign. Centralization is what you want and peripheralization is what you want to avoid.

Because in the majority of cases overall, extension (backward bending) of the spine is the most beneficial position in reducing or centralizing pain, McKenzie exercises are often called "McKenzie extension exercises". In the case of spinal stenosis though, symptoms caused by posterior element issues often respond best to flexion (forward bending). Because different cases respond differently to the various positions, true McKenzie Method actually tests for the position(s) that are beneficial for an individual patient. So, depending on your particular circumstances, you will usually wind up using one of 6 positions: flexion, extension, or left or right side bending combined with flexion or extension – depending on what position best reduces or centralizes symptoms.

As with the McKenzie Method for the cervical spine, central and/or intervertebral stenosis caused primarily by a disc protrusion will usually respond best to one of the extension positions, so I recommend you test those first if you know that a disc protrusion is a significant factor in your case. If one of those positions does prove effective, there is no need to test the flexion positions.

On the other hand, intervertebral stenosis caused primarily by posterior element conditions (bone spurring/thickening and/or ligament thickening/buckling) will usually respond best to flexion, so those positions should be tested first in those circumstances.

In cases where both disc and posterior element factors are producing the stenosis, it may be necessary to alternate one or more of the flexion and extension positions. In this situation, test all positions and begin by using whichever worked the best (in centralizing or reducing symptoms). If at some point that position is no longer helpful or actually seems to increase symptoms, re-test and change to the new best position you find. This process of switching positions will likely continue for some time if you are having stenosis from both the front and back portions of the effected spinal canal(s).

The following pictures illustrate the positions for the lumbar spine that should be tested and compared to determine the position that best centralizes symptoms:

The McKenzie Method Lumbar Spine Positions

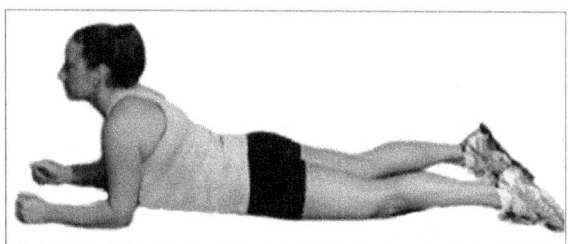

Straight extension: *Begin by lying on your stomach on a firm surface and then raise up, propping yourself on your elbows as shown. Hold this position for 30 seconds to a minute and note any changes in your symptoms to compare the degree of centralization (reduction of symptoms furthest from the spine) or symptom improvement (if your symptoms were localized near the spine to begin with) to the other positions you test. Occasionally, there will be an initial peripheralization or increase in symptoms when getting into position, so allow 30 seconds or so before assessing the amount of centralization or symptom improvement.*

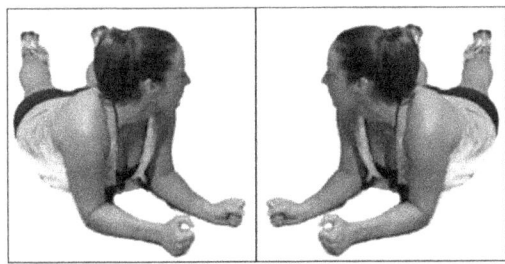

Extension with left and right side bending: *(note, you will only use left OR right side-bending if it was better than straight extension). Begin by lying on your stomach on a firm surface and then raise up, propping yourself on your elbows and then shifting your upper body to the side as shown. Hold this position for 30 seconds to a minute and note any changes in your symptoms to compare the degree of centralization (reduction of symptoms furthest from the spine) or symptom improvement (if your symptoms were localized near the spine to begin with) to the other positions you test. Return to the straight extension position and then shift to the opposite side to test that position. Occasionally, there will be an initial peripheralization or increase in symptoms when getting into position, so allow 30 seconds or so before assessing the amount of centralization or symptom improvement.*

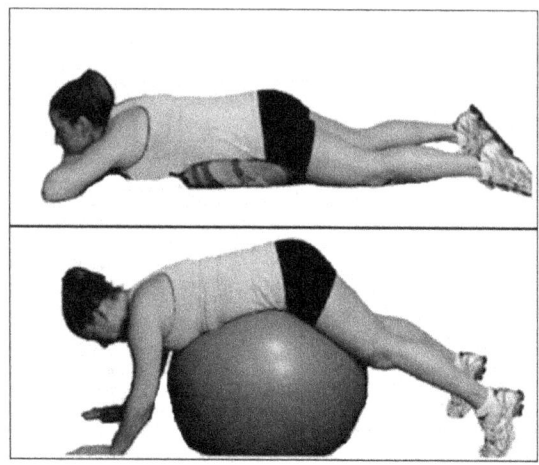

Flexion: *(an exercise ball works best, but for testing purposes, a pillow or stack of pillows under the abdomen will work. Simply lie face down with the ball or pillows under your stomach and relax your abdominal muscles. Hold this position for 30 seconds to a minute and note any changes in your symptoms to compare the degree of centralization (reduction of symptoms furthest from the spine) or symptom improvement (if your symptoms were localized near the spine to begin with) to the other positions you test.*

If straight flexion is helpful, flexion combined with left and right side bending should also be tested, but these positions are rarely used and because they can dramatically irritate disc-related symptoms these positions are not shown. Again, they should only be tested if straight flexion is helpful.

To repeat, you may have some pain when you first move into a new position. After you get into each position, wait 30 seconds to a minute to see what happens with your symptoms. The thing to remember is that you are looking for a position that eases the symptoms the furthest away from the spine first. For example, if you have pain running down the back of your leg all the way to the foot, a good position would be one that moves the pain out of the foot and calf, even if it intensifies pain in the buttocks or low back. If you only had symptoms in the buttock and thigh, a good position would be one that moves the pain out of the buttock and thigh, even if it gets worse in the low back.

If there is no clear "winner" as a position that best centralizes your symptoms, begin with using the straight extension position.

Any position that causes peripheralization of the symptoms –that is, makes the symptoms the furthest from the spine WORSE or causes symptoms to extend further from the spine - should be avoided!

In other words, do NOT continue with any position that makes symptoms either more intense in the leg or extend further down the leg.

If every position causes increased symptoms at the furthest point from the spine, and/or causes the symptoms to extend further down the leg from the spine, DO NOT perform any of the McKenzie exercises (in such cases, professional evaluation and treatment is strongly recommended!).

Otherwise, keep testing different positions until you find the one that does the best job of alleviating the symptoms furthest from the spine. Once you find the position that works the best, hold that position for 1 to 2 minutes and then take a break for 30 seconds or so in a neutral position. Repeat the beneficial position frequently (try to do it at least once or twice every hour you are awake and up to five or six times is even better), as long as it continues to relieve the symptoms furthest from the spine. With doing the exercise frequently, you may develop some soreness in the muscles of the back. Most people gladly accept some soreness in exchange for relief of more severe symptoms, but if you are bothered by it, simply reduce the frequency of the exercise somewhat and it will usually subside on its own within a day or so. Alternately, some massage of the sore areas will usually alleviate it pretty quickly.

Note, you will only be using the ONE position that gives you the best centralization of symptoms.

You will not be using any of the other positions unless you reach a point where the chosen position no longer provides further centralization after 3 or more days of frequent use. If this occurs, re-test to see if a different position works better.

As mentioned earlier, if you know you have a disc protrusion as a primary cause of your symptoms, in most cases one of the extension positions (straight extension, extension with left side-bending, or extension with right side-bending) will be the most effective. If that is the case with you, the following modification will usually enhance the benefits of the extension exercise:

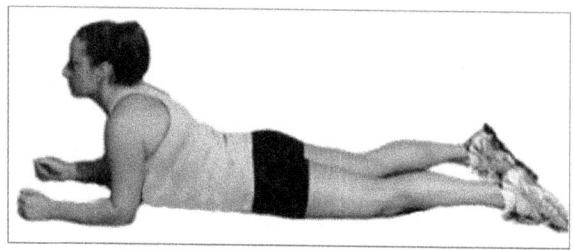

Begin as usual with the McKenzie exercise by propping yourself up on your elbows (and bend left or right if one of these positions improved your results with the Basic McKenzie Method).

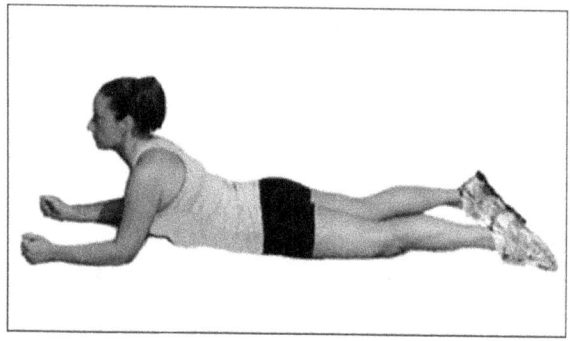

Next, shift your elbows forward an inch or two, as shown above.

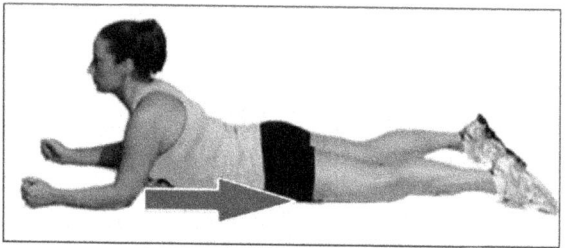

Finally, pull back with your arms, so that your upper body is pulled forward. Do not pull so hard that your lower body slides, but enough that you can feel a pull on the pelvis. This produces a mild traction on the low back and this traction combined with the spinal extension can be quite effective.

As an alternative to the lying flat on the floor version of spinal extension, you can achieve similar effects with spinal extension done on your hands and knees as shown below:

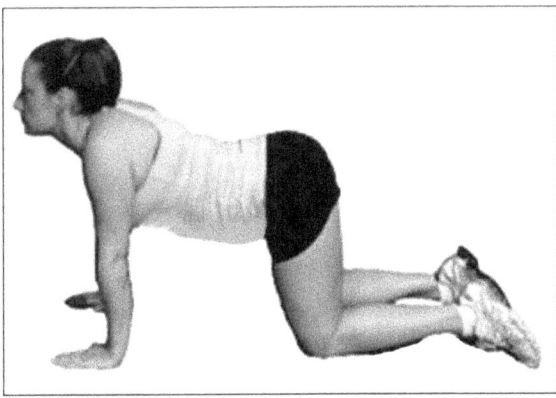

Modified Extension: *Simply allow the abdomen to hang down so that the spine curves towards the floor.*

Lumbosacral / Hip Flexibility and Alignment

There are numerous stretches and flexibility exercises that can be done. The recommended exercises have been kept to a minimum here for two reasons. First, it is the author's experience that people will tend to stick with a short, simple exercise regimen far better than a complicated one with many exercises. A simple exercise regimen done regularly is far more beneficial than a complicated one that doesn't get done.

The other reason that the author has limited the number of exercises presented is due to the fact that, as you've seen, spinal stenosis is due to different factors, and while one person may respond very well to a given exercise, a different person might actually worsen as a result of doing certain exercises. The exercises presented in this book are well-tolerated by the vast majority of people with spinal stenosis (but there are exceptions, so if an exercise seems to worsen your symptoms, don't do it!). If you wish to use different or additional exercises that you have found to be helpful, by all means do them!

The flexibility exercises that follow will work best when done a few times throughout the day (rather than one long period of exercises, two to four short sessions per day is recommended). They can be used during times of major symptoms, but it is usually best to focus more on doing the McKenzie exercise that best centralizes your symptoms during those times and then transitioning more to the flexibility and alignment exercises (along with the McKenzie exercise) one or two times per day for prevention when the symptoms are less intense or absent.

In some cases, major symptoms can be produced by tight muscles, so the flexibility exercises are definitely worth a try if you are not getting satisfactory results from the McKenzie exercise alone.

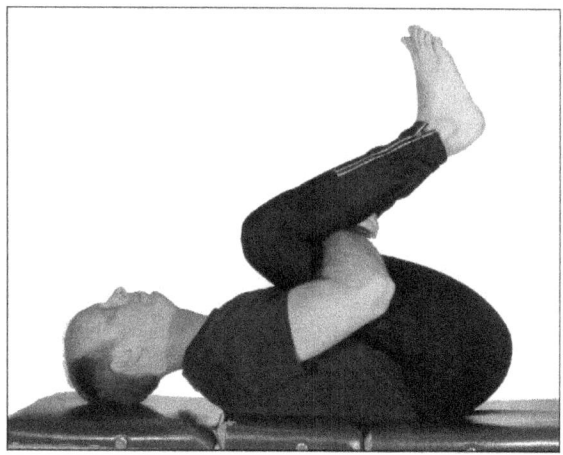

Knee to Chest: *Place your hands behind your knees (to prevent undue stress on the knee joints). Take a breath in and let it out as you pull your thighs tightly to your chest. Hold for 15 to 30 seconds and release as you breathe in. Repeat two or more times (as your time allows).*

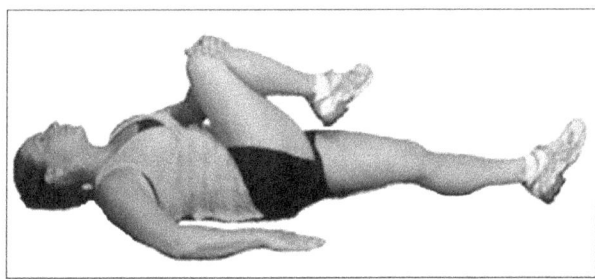

Piriformis Stretch: *Begin by lying on your back and firmly but gently pulling your knee towards your chest. When you have the leg as far up as you can go, pull it across your body toward the opposite shoulder. Hold for 15 to 30 seconds and repeat two or more times with each leg - even if you only have symptoms on one side, it is best to stretch both sides.*

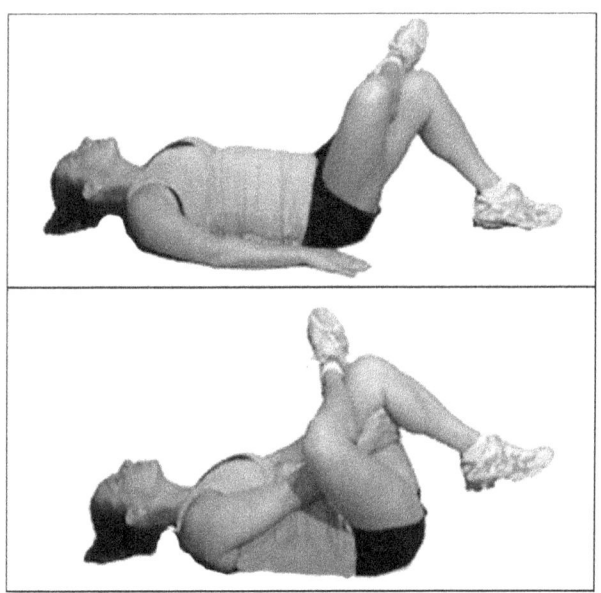

Figure 4 Stretch (For the Gluteus Minimus): *Lie on your back with your legs bent and cross one leg over the other, resting the ankle just above the knee of the supporting leg. Reach behind the supporting leg with your hands and pull the thigh towards your chest. Try to keep the knee of the crossed leg pointing out to the side as much as possible as you pull the supporting leg towards your chest. You should feel a pull in the buttock of the crossed leg. Hold the stretch for 15 to 30 seconds and then switch legs. Stretch each leg two or more times (as your time allows).*

Low Back Stabilization

Many people with back problems assume that they have weak back muscles, but in most cases (except in people de-conditioned by extended bed rest), the back muscles themselves are quite strong and the weaknesses actually lie in the "core" muscles of the abdomen and/or the leg and buttock muscles. The exercises that follow provide basic conditioning for these groups of muscles. Again, these exercises are intended more for prevention and maintenance rather than during times of major symptoms, but they sometimes do help reduce symptoms and are worth trying for symptom relief as well.

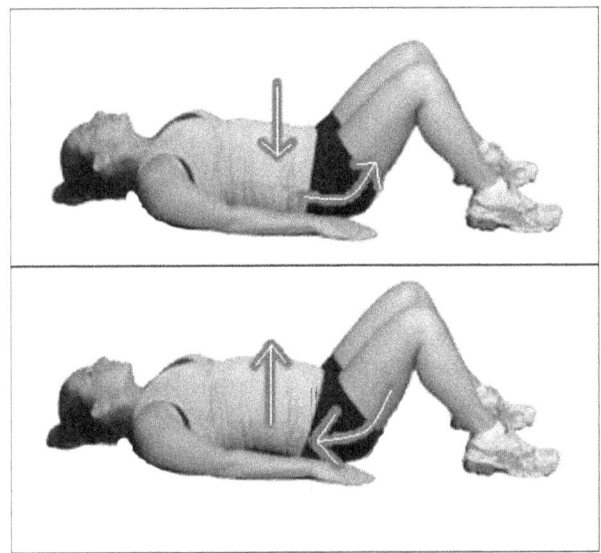

Basic Pelvic Tilt: *Lie on your back with your knees bent. In the relaxed position, there should be a small space between your low back and the surface you are lying on. Contract your stomach muscles and press your lower back towards the surface as you rock your pelvis down and towards your feet as shown in the top image. Hold for 10 seconds and then relax, allowing your lower back to rise slightly and your pelvis to rock back to the starting position (as shown in the bottom image). Repeat 10 to 30 times (or more if you wish to do so, but start with 10 to 30 the first few times to be sure the exercise does not aggravate your symptoms).*

If you have stenosis due to a disc protrusion, you may find it helpful to add a step to the exercise by going beyond the relaxed position and contracting your lower back muscles, tilting your pelvis the opposite direction, and accentuating the curve in the low back (increasing the space between your low back and the floor as compared to the relaxed position). When doing this variation, you would hold each end position for 10 seconds, relaxing briefly in between. As with the regular version, repeat 10 to 30 times.

Once you feel comfortable with the movement of the basic pelvic tilt, it is recommended that you transition to the advanced pelvic tilt exercise that follows.

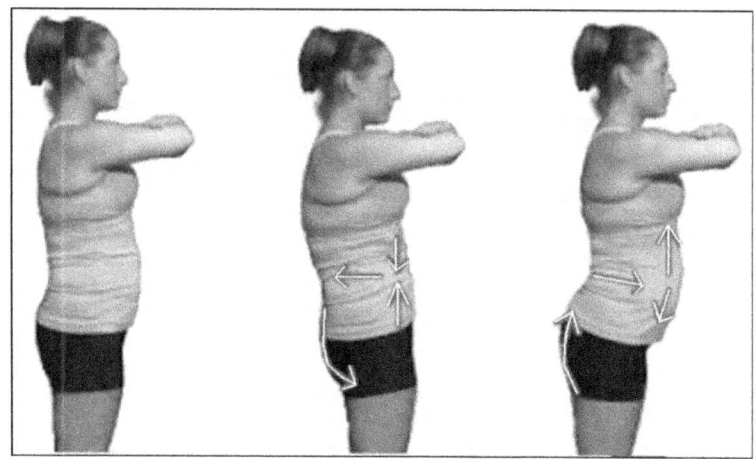

Advanced Pelvic Tilt: *Stand straight and begin by contacting your abdominal muscles and rocking your pelvis back and downward, flattening your low back. Hold for 10 seconds. Next, relax your abdominal muscles and rock your pelvis up and forward, allowing the curve to return to the low back.*

As with the Basic Pelvic Tilt, if you have a lumbar disc protrusion, you may find it helpful to go beyond the relaxed position and contract the back muscles and rock the pelvis up and forward even more to accentuate the forward curve in the lumbar spine.

With either version, hold the contracted position(s) for 10 seconds and relax momentarily between the contracted positions. Repeat 10 to 30 times (or more, if you like).

*Tip – If you have trouble getting the movement down initially when transitioning from the Basic Pelvic Tilt, try doing the Advanced Pelvic Tilt standing with your back against a wall at first, so you can feel your back's position against the wall as you get used to the movements.

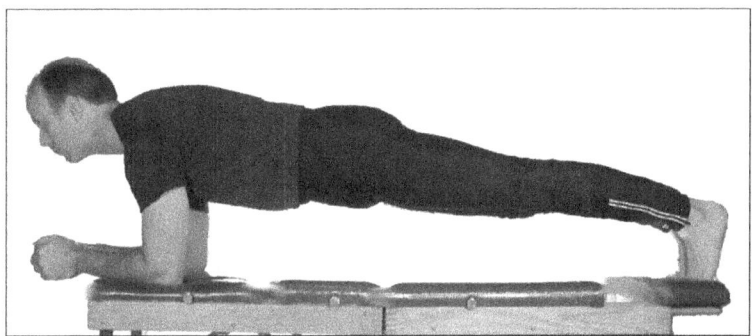

Planks: *Planks are one of the simplest, yet most effective exercises for strengthening the abdominal core muscles. There are many variations, but you don't really need to get fancy with them. The basic version above works quite well for most people.*

Start by lying on your stomach and rise up on your elbows and toes as shown, keeping your back straight. Try to hold the position for at least 30 seconds and gradually work up to 2 minutes or more over a period of days or weeks. Two or more sessions per day (of 30 seconds to 2 minutes each) is recommended.

If your abdominal muscles are very weak, you may not be able to do 30 seconds, or may not be able to even get into the full plank position at all, in which case you may wish to start with the modified version that follows.

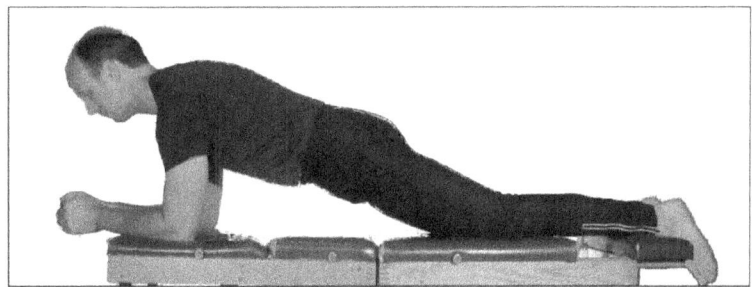

Modified Planks: *Start by lying on your stomach and then raise up on your elbows, keeping your back straight and your lower legs relaxed as shown above. Try to hold the position for at least 30 seconds and work up to at least one minute before switching to the regular plank exercise shown previously.*

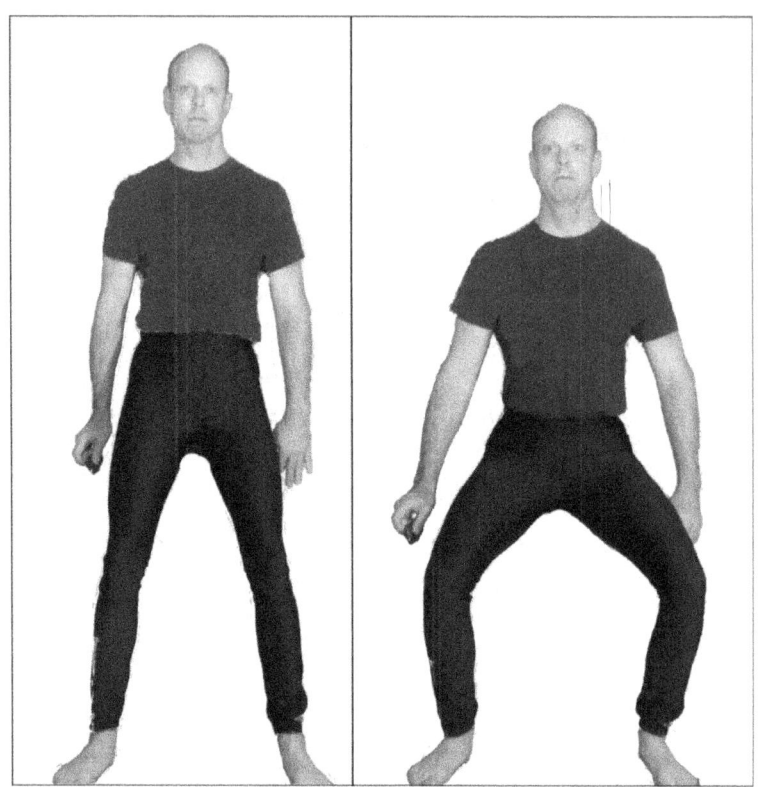

Wall Squats: *This is a basic exercise for strengthening the muscles of the thighs and buttocks. There are many other exercises that can be done to strengthen these muscles and if you have found different one or more different exercises that you prefer, feel free to use those instead.*

Start by standing with your back against a wall with your feet shoulder width apart and approximately 12 to 18 inches out from the wall (the taller you are, the further your feet need to be out from the wall). Be sure that your feet will not slip on the floor before attempting the exercise. Slowly slide your back down the wall, bending your knees as you lower yourself. Try to get down to where your knees are bent to 90 degrees (your thighs are parallel to the floor), but if you cannot due to knee problems or weakness, just get as low as you can. Hold the lowered position for 30 seconds to a minute, or as long as you can. Slide back up to the upright standing position, relax for a moment and repeat 2 to 3 times (or more, if you like).

Chapter 13: Inversion / Home Traction

Inversion and/or traction are sometimes beneficial for stenosis from disc protrusion and/or posterior element (joint and ligament) thickening alike. The long-axis stretching inversion/traction places on the spine may reduce disc bulging and can stretch the ligaments and muscles surrounding the areas of stenosis to reduce narrowing of nerve passages and alleviate symptoms caused by secondary muscle contraction.

Unfortunately, inversion or traction can also trigger increased inflammation and muscle spasm during the acute stage of symptoms. For this reason, the author generally recommends these treatments more for prevention and the alleviation of mild symptoms after the acute inflammatory stage has passed. Even so, some people do get relief of acute symptoms with inversion and traction, so it is an option in such situations. If you do decide to try such treatment while major symptoms are present, it is strongly recommended that you proceed with caution. In addition, whenever beginning with inversion therapy, it is a good idea to have someone present to assist you in getting on and off the inversion table and to otherwise provide assistance if you react unfavorably to it.

Generally speaking, inversion is better suited to treating lumbar conditions than cervical conditions. Conversely, home traction devices for the cervical spine (neck) are usually more effective and easier to set up than those intended for the lumbar spine (low back).

Inversion Devices

There are many inversion products out there, and they vary considerably in cost and quality. While it may be tempting to purchase one of the cheaper inversion devices, it is extremely important to invest in a good-quality product. The last thing anyone with spinal stenosis needs is to have their inversion machine collapse underneath them or drop them on their head.

Because quality is important, the author recommends the Teeter line of inversion tables (but not their inversion boots, as I'll discuss shortly).

Teeter's inversion tables are UL listed, meaning they've been tested by the independent Underwriters Laboratories and found to be safe for their intended use. Most inversion equipment has not been subjected to independent safety testing. While this does not mean that other tables are unsafe, the author is more confident in recommending Teeter because of their UL listing.

Most Teeter tables are rated for people up to 300 pounds, so it should go without saying, but if you're well over 300 pounds, DON'T USE THIS EQUIPMENT!

Another thing to consider is that the Teeter equipment is designed for people up to 6'6", which is a pretty generous amount of head space. But if you happen to be taller than 6'6", this is not a good product for you.

Finally, because of the fact that inversion will alter blood pressure going to the head, if you have any history of dizziness, stroke, or loss of consciousness, be sure to check with your doctor before investing in an inversion table. Even if you have never had any such problems, it is strongly advised that you start out slowly with inversion, and begin with the one of the lesser degrees of inversion (most Teeter inversion tables have settings for 20 degrees, 60 degrees, and 90 degrees) for brief periods of time. For example, on your first inversion session, the author suggests starting at just 20 degrees and staying there for 30 seconds to a minute at a time to test how your body reacts. If all goes well, first increase the time at 20 degrees - perhaps a few minutes at a time. If things are still going well after a few days at 20 degrees, then you may wish to increase to 60 degrees, but back off on the time again (to about 30 second to a minute the first time) for the first few sessions.

For many people, 60 degrees is plenty of inversion to get the results they want and is much more comfortable than 90 degrees, so if you're happy with the way thing are going at 60 degrees, there really is no need to go to the 90 degree setting. If you do decide to try the 90 degree setting, it is strongly recommended that you have another person present the first few times to help you, in case you experience any problems.

Not Recommended: Inversion Boots

There are three main reasons I don't recommend inversion boots, whether they are made by Teeter or any other company. The first reason is that, unlike inversion tables, there's only one option for the amount of inversion. It's all or nothing, and this can put you at risk of various problems related to the increased blood flow to the head, or increase your stenosis-related symptoms. Just getting into position to use inversion boots is physically challenging and is probably not a good idea for someone with a history of back problems.

The second reason I'm not a fan of inversion boots is the safety (or lack of safety) issue. Most inversion boots are used to hang upside down in a doorway from some type of bracket system. Even the best of brackets can come loose for one reason or another, and that results in you suddenly getting dropped on your head - not good!

Finally, even we ignore the first two reasons, there have been some issues with the development of joint instability problems, particularly in the ankles and knees, in inversion boot users. Not only does inversion stretch the back, but when you're doing it by hanging from inversion boots, it also stretches the ligaments in the ankles and knees. With the full, unsupported inversion that you get with inversion boots, the stretch on these ligaments can often be more than they are designed to handle, and the result is unstable joints that are susceptible to injury.

Basically, if you want to do inversion, stick with a good quality inversion table which has straps that support you from your pelvis/hips and does not place stress on your ankles and knees.

Home Traction Devices:

Again, it has been the author's experience that inversion is more effective and easier to use for lumbar (low back) conditions whereas home traction devices are more effective for cervical (neck) spinal stenosis. There are some good lumbar traction devices that are suitable for home use, but they tend to be expensive (as much or more than a good quality inversion table) and usually require some training from a professional familiar with their use before attempting to use one on your own at home. For these reasons, the discussion that follows is focused on traction devices for the neck that are generally easy to use and don't require significant formal instruction on how to use them.

There is a wide variety of cervical traction devices for home use, ranging from over-the-door pulley and weight systems, to devices you lie down on and strap your head into, to collars that you pump air into to expand them and stretch your neck. Generally, the more complicated a cervical traction device is to set up and use, the less effective it is in the long run because it typically won't be used as often as it needs to be for best results.

In terms of effectiveness, the devices that are used lying down (such as the ComforTrac or the Saunders Cervical Home Trac) are usually the best, assuming that the head cradle is the right fit for your head. Lying down allows better relaxation of the supporting muscles of the neck so that the traction doesn't have as much resistance to overcome. Most of these traction units have some sort of hand pump that adjusts the traction force and a button or lever to release the air pressure to discontinue the traction. Unfortunately, this type of traction device is usually significantly more expensive than other types, with a price tag of a few hundred dollars being typical for a well-made unit.

A more budget-friendly, yet still relatively effective and easy to use option is one of the inflatable collar types of cervical traction. These can usually be used either upright or lying down, although the shape of them requires some creative pillow positioning to comfortably use them when lying down. This type of traction device also has the advantage that it can be used when moving around, so they can be used frequently without a lot of disruption in other activities. Even so, whenever possible, it's best to try to take a few minutes and relax while doing the traction so that there is less muscle resistance to the treatment. Decent quality units of this type (such as those by ChiSoft or Instapark) are available in the $30 to $50 range.

The over-the-door traction devices that use weights and pulleys to provide the pull are the cheapest of the bunch (available for $20 or less), but that low price comes with several disadvantages. They are the most complicated to set up of the traction devices intended for home use. They often have uncomfortable head harnesses that have been known to actually cause TMJ disorders. They require you to stay in one place and are the most difficult to get out of if you need to move quickly for some reason. They take up space and are unsightly on whatever door you set them up on. In short, they're just not very good. At one time, over-the-door pulley devices were the only thing available for home cervical traction, but there really isn't a good reason to use this type of device anymore when there are better options available for a little bit more money.

Some home traction devices have some sort of indicator to tell you how much traction force you are applying and some do not. In a clinical setting, knowing the traction force is useful for documentation purposes and for measuring progress. In the home treatment environment, it's far less important. The thing to keep in mind is that the traction force applied should be relatively comfortable. Using higher force is not desirable if it is causing you discomfort because your muscles will begin to tense and resist the treatment. The result of using too much force is usually increased symptoms, not faster recovery. Feeling a pull or stretch is good. Feeling pain is not. As you get adapted to traction, you will likely apply more traction force to get to the stretch. This is to be expected as the structures being tractioned will relax and loosen up. As long as you stick to a traction intensity that produces a stretch without significant pain (having a few minor twinges when your first start applying the traction is acceptable), you should do fine.

When starting out with traction, it's best to begin with short intervals. A minute or two at a time is a good starting point to be sure that the traction is not going to aggravate your symptoms. As you get accustomed to using traction, you can gradually increase your time if you like. Ten to fifteen minutes at a time is usually plenty for a single session, although some authors recommend up to 30 minutes per session. It is the author's experience that most people get the best results by doing short sessions frequently, rather than one or two long sessions. For example, provided the patient can work it into their schedule, it usually works better to do three 10 minute sessions per day than one 30 minute session.

Chapter 14: Lifestyle Modifications

Diet:

Diet can have a dramatic effect on symptoms by means of biochemical effects on inflammation and muscle contraction. The focus of this book is on improving symptoms related to spinal stenosis and for the sake of simplicity, recommendations regarding diet will be made without an in-depth discussion of the biochemistry and physiology behind those recommendations. In addition, while there are numerous possible dietary changes that may be helpful, the author has stuck with basic recommendations that will give maximum benefit from relatively simple changes. In the long run it is best to adopt the recommendations that follow into your usual dietary habits, but they are particularly important during times of increased symptoms.

The first, and probably most important recommendation is to minimize the consumption of grain-based foods and refined sugars. Whole grains are nutritionally better than refined grains, but for the purposes of reducing spinal stenosis symptoms, it's best to minimize consumption of all grains. These foods tend to increase inflammation to some degree in most people, and can dramatically increase inflammation in sensitive individuals. If you absolutely can't live without eating grains, gluten-free products are recommended.

Sugar sneaks into the diet in many ways, and many times people are unaware of the amount of sugar they are consuming. One of the biggest sources of refined sugar in the diet in developed countries is soft drinks. An average 12 ounce soft drink contains 35 to 45 grams of sugar, which is equivalent to 8 to 10 teaspoons! For many people, simply cutting out or reducing soft drink consumption will significantly reduce their inflammation-related symptoms.   Other foods and beverages that tend to have a surprisingly high sugar content are white breads, cereals, flavored yogurts, juice drinks, and energy drinks, so minimizing consumption of these products is strongly recommended.

Sugar substitutes (NutraSweet, Equal, Splenda, etc.) are actually not a good replacement for sugar when it comes to controlling inflammation. In fact, given the choice between an artificial sweetener and a small quantity of sugar, sugar is probably the better choice for most individuals. Of the sweeteners available, from an inflammation standpoint, honey (when used in moderation), is probably the best option in most cases.

The next recommendation is to maximize the intake of fresh vegetables. If fresh vegetables are not readily available, frozen is a reasonably good second-choice. In addition to generally being anti-inflammatory in nature, many vegetables contain nutrients that the body needs for tissue repair and regeneration. In addition, for those concerned that a diet low in grains will result in too little dietary fiber, that issue is solved by eating lots of vegetables. There are a few vegetables that may increase inflammation in some situations, primarily the nightshade plants such as tomatoes, eggplant, and peppers, and consumption of these foods is best kept to a minimum, especially when significant symptoms are present.

When it comes to meats, the more natural, the better. Wild-caught fish, free-range chicken, and grass-fed beef have a more favorable balance of fats in them for keeping inflammation in check than their "regular" farm raised counterparts. A large part of inflammation control has to do with the balance of Omega-6 fats to Omega-3 fats. From an inflammation control standpoint, it's best to have a ratio of somewhere around 1:1 to 5:1 of Omega-6 to Omega-3. The typical American diet is usually in excess of 20:1. This is largely due to our high direct consumption of grains, but also due to eating meats that were raised on grain-based feeds.

As you might have guessed from the discussion on the ratio of Omega-6 to Omega-3 fats in meats, choosing the right fats and oils for cooking and other means of consumption can also help control inflammation. Most vegetable oils and margarines contain primarily omega-6 fats and their use should be kept to a minimum. Olive oil, coconut oil, and butter, when consumed in moderation, are the best (of the readily-available practical options) to avoid promoting inflammation.

Avoid Smoking:

It's no secret that smoking is unhealthy, but most people think in terms of smoking's negative effects on the respiratory and cardiovascular systems. Smoking is also associated with chronic back pain and is thought to contribute to degenerative joint disease. In addition to promoting inflammation, smoking decreases circulation and the supply of oxygen to the tissues and interferes with regeneration and healing.

Hydration:

If the section on diet has you thinking about replacing your soft drink consumption with a less damaging alternative, water (uncarbonated, unflavored water) is the best way to go! Chronic dehydration is thought to contribute to degeneration of the spinal discs, as well as to muscle and joint pain.

The amount of water you should consume depends on several factors and there really isn't a "one-size-fits-all" quantity you should drink, but for the sake of simplicity, the usual eight 8 ounce glasses per day recommendation is not likely to do any harm, and will put most people into the right ballpark.

To more accurately monitor your hydration, there are relatively inexpensive test strips available to measure hydration, but you can also get a good indication simply by looking at the color of your urine. If the color of your urine is faint, your hydration is reasonably good. If it's distinctly yellow, you should drink more water. Bear in mind that these basic color rules don't apply if you are taking a lot of vitamin supplements (particularly those containing B-complex vitamins), or medications that are known to alter urine color.

Activity/General Exercise:

In addition to exercises specifically directed at areas involved in your spinal stenosis, it is extremely helpful to be physically active and to get some general-purpose exercise daily, or at least every other day. With spinal stenosis of all types and causes, it's best to stick with low-impact exercise and resistance training that does not put undue pressure on the affected areas of the spine. Walking, swimming, bicycling (both actual bicycling and on a stationary bike), and elliptical training are all good options for general-purpose exercise.

Weight/resistance training is also useful, but it is extremely important to maintain good form and to avoid certain exercises that may cause or aggravate problems depending on the nature of your stenosis.

In cases where disc protrusion is a factor, it is best to avoid any exercise that requires you to bend forward at the waist while standing or sitting, unless your torso is somehow supported. For example, straight-leg deadlifts and "Good Mornings" are a bad idea, as are rows done without any support for the chest, but crunches on an ab machine or rows on machines with a chest support are fine - as long as you use good form with appropriate resistance for your strength.

If you have significant posterior element stenosis, it's best to avoid exercises that require you to bend backwards at the waist. For example, the back extension machine and "kick-backs" are usually best avoided in this situation.

Stretching and floor exercises such as yoga or Pilates are mostly fine to do as a whole regardless of the type of stenosis, but certain positions are best to be avoided in some cases. Here again, the basic rule of thumb is to use caution with or avoid poses/exercises that put the spine into flexion (forward bending) with disc-related stenosis, and use caution with or avoid poses and exercises that place the spine in extension (backward bending) with posterior element stenosis.

Chapter 15: Professional Treatment Options

A Word About Health Care Providers

The majority of health care providers are well-trained and well-intentioned men and women who really want to help their patients. That being said, there are those in every profession who are less concerned about the needs of the people they serve than their own needs and desires. Even those who are extremely dedicated to their patients are sometimes led astray by their egos and biases when it comes to making treatment decisions and recommendations. For this reason the author suggests that if you have any doubts about the recommendations a health care provider gives you, seek another opinion.

While in most cases of spinal stenosis, achieving complete, immediate symptom relief is unlikely regardless of treatment, most patients will have some noticeable improvement within a few weeks when the treatment is working. Although ups and downs in symptoms are common from one day to the next, the overall trend for every two to three week period should be toward improvement (unless there is an intervening situation that interferes, such as a new trauma or unusual stress). If this is not occurring, re-evaluation is usually warranted to decide if a change in treatment approach is needed. Even the best of health care providers can get caught up in carrying out a preconceived treatment plan and may not fully realize when things aren't going according to that plan. You may need to prompt your health care provider to re-evaluate when things aren't improving as expected, and if they seem unwilling to do so without a good explanation as to why, you may need to consider changing providers.

Depending on the nature and severity of your particular situation, complete symptom resolution may not be possible regardless of treatment. Your health care provider may not be forthcoming about this initially because a positive mental attitude toward treatment is thought to help patients achieve better outcomes. So, if your doctor initially gives you high hopes and then later backtracks on what might or might not be possible in your case, he or she may not have been maliciously misleading you, but simply trying to get you the best outcome possible.

Non-Invasive Treatments

Spinal Manipulation

Spinal manipulation is a treatment used most often by doctors of chiropractic, but also by osteopathic doctors, some physical therapists and massage therapists, and a few medical doctors. The basic concept of spinal manipulation is to find areas of abnormal spinal alignment or motion and correct them (as much as possible) using either manual thrusts, stretching/positioning techniques, or various instruments to direct focused force into the spine.

Correcting spinal alignment and motion has several effects, the most important of which may be changing the firing pattern of nerve receptors in the spinal joints and surrounding tissues to better allow the central nervous system to monitor and control things such as muscle contraction and coordination and circulation. Patients are often surprised at how quickly pain can be alleviated with manipulation techniques, which in some cases occurs almost immediately.

Many people are initially fearful of spinal manipulation, but a skilled practitioner is usually well-versed in a variety of methods for providing the desired correction safely and without undue pain or discomfort to the patient. In the case of particularly fearful patients, or in cases where bone fragility is a potential issue (due to osteoporosis or other abnormalities of the bones), low-force methods may be used at least initially, such as Activator (for information, visit www.Activator.com), Arthrostim (www.impacinc.net), or Sigma Methods (www.sigmamethods.com). These low-force techniques use various instruments that deliver high-speed tapping to the joints to lightly coax them into alignment and to improve mobility.

Regardless of the technique used, in most cases, the best and most lasting results from spinal manipulation will come with repeated treatments over time. How many treatments it takes to get maximum results varies tremendously depending on the specific situation, but as a general rule, noticeable improvement will occur within a few weeks in most cases. Although most people will begin to feel better within a few sessions, some individuals experience post-treatment soreness early on in the treatment regimen. Such soreness is usually mild and typically ceases after a few treatment sessions.

Many chiropractors and other practitioners who utilize spinal manipulation will also provide other physical medicine services, which will be discussed in the sections on Massage, Physical Therapy, and Acupuncture.

Massage

Although the underlying cause of the symptoms in spinal stenosis is nerve compression and irritation, the direct symptoms often come from reactions in the muscles. In some cases, these muscle reactions take on a life of their own and may remain even after the nerve issues are alleviated. One of the best ways for dealing with muscle related symptoms is massage therapy.

In particular, "myofascial release" and "deep tissue" techniques can dramatically reduce symptoms and improve mobility in cases of spinal stenosis. These methods can be somewhat uncomfortable at times while they are being performed, but they loosen constricted muscles and improve circulation, providing symptom relief that can last for days or weeks. In cases where there is significant ongoing nerve irritation, the effects of massage tend to be shorter-lived, but even then it can make symptoms much more tolerable.

One concern that people often have about massage therapy is that they will have to get undressed. Professional licensed massage therapists always drape their clients with a sheet or blanket to maintain modesty, and most can work around some clothing if you are uncomfortable with disrobing. If this is a concern for you, it is strongly recommended that you discuss the matter with prospective massage therapists before scheduling an appointment, so that both you and the therapist are on the same page and you can better relax for your treatment. If you don't feel comfortable with a particular massage therapist in advance of your session, you will likely do better to choose a different one, as trust and relaxation are important to getting the best therapeutic result.

Physical Therapy

Physical therapy is a profession, not a treatment, and there is a wide variety of treatments that may be used by a physical therapist (or other professional licensed to perform physical therapy modalities, such as a doctor of chiropractic, medical doctor, etc.). Because of this, it is recommended that if you do "go to PT", that you ask about the specific treatments being used. This information can be useful in the event that you wind up seeing a different health care practitioner and he or she wants to know what treatments worked and what didn't (as this information is useful in both diagnosis and in making further treatment decisions). Although most experienced health care practitioners can kind of figure out patient descriptions of treatments like "that electro-shock thing that made my muscles tingle", or the "telephone thingy they rubbed the lotion in with", you being able to describe the treatments by their actual names can come in handy. Of course, practitioners new to working with you will request records from your previous treatment providers, but there can be a delay in actually receiving those records, so the information you provide can speed up the process of you getting effective treatment with the new provider.

When significant symptoms are present, most physical therapists will begin with what are known collectively as passive modalities. Passive refers to the fact that the treatments are done to you, with little to no action on your part other than to show up for the treatment session. Such treatment modalities include various types of electrical stimulation, therapeutic ultrasound (which is very different from diagnostic ultrasound), massage, heat or cold packs, and laser therapy. These modalities are all primarily intended to reduce symptoms by means of either direct nerve sedation and muscle relaxation, or by means of altering circulation.

Once major symptoms are decreasing, physical therapists will usually transition into active modalities. Active means that you are now participating in the treatment. Active therapy includes things like stretching and strengthening exercises, balance and coordination training, and gait training. These treatments are intended to provide a more lasting improvement in your condition by means of correcting muscle imbalances, improving mobility, and providing stabilization to damaged structures.

Although most physical therapists recommend preventive use of the various exercises and active treatment methods to their patients when they release them from ongoing treatment, many patients (probably the majority) fail to follow such recommendations. This is not entirely the fault of the patients, though. In many cases, the critical importance of continued use of exercises and other treatments to prevent a return of symptoms is not adequately communicated. There is a tendency for patients to think that once their symptoms are gone, they are "cured", and this is rarely the case.

When you stop doing exercises, you lose the beneficial effects of those exercises. **So, to be very clear on this, if you got better doing certain exercises, you need to continue doing those exercises – probably for the rest of your life!** The only exception to this rule is in cases where you were doing unevenly loaded exercises to correct some sort of imbalance. For example, if you had a postural distortion where the resting position of your head had it turned slightly to one side, a physical therapist might have you exercise the muscles unevenly to straighten out your head. Once such an imbalance is corrected, you would of course discontinue the unevenly loaded exercise, otherwise, you'd eventually create the opposite imbalance.

The importance of continuing effective active therapy once you are released from formal treatment brings up a second issue. In many cases, all of a person's active therapy was done using specialized machines that most people do not have convenient access to. For this reason, the author recommends that if you do go through a program of physical therapy, you should work with your therapist (well in advance of your release from care) to devise a program you can do on your own at home or at a gym to maintain the gains you achieve in treatment.

Portable Electrical Stimulators

Although more of a self-treatment measure, TENS units, portable muscle stimulators, and microcurrent stimulator devices are available most often by prescription from a licensed health care provider (although a very simple version is currently being marketed by the makers of Icy Hot). Their use is contraindicated for patients with pacemakers and other implanted electrical devices.

These devices are scaled-down battery-powered versions of the electrical stimulation devices used by physical therapists, chiropractors, and physical medicine doctors. There are some differences in the output currents and physiological effects of the different portable stimulators.

TENS (Transcutaneous Electrical Nerve Stimulation) units are primarily for blocking pain. The basic theory is that the TENS unit emits a frequency that activates the transmission of signals through nerves that block the perception of pain signals in the central nervous system. Many people find that a TENS unit provides as much or more symptom relief than pain medication, and is much less likely to cause significant side-effects. Although many people get good results from the default settings on TENS units right out of the box, some individuals will need to have the setting adjusted by an experienced professional to get optimal results.

Electrical muscle stimulators (also called EMS units) work by means of causing muscle contractions with the intent of fatiguing tight muscles and forcing them to relax. Some people find these devices helpful, but in the author's experience this type of device appears to be the least effective overall of the portable electrical stimulator devices for reducing symptoms for spinal stenosis sufferers.

Microcurrent stimulators (sometimes referred to as MENS units), use a very low-level electrical current that is usually imperceptible to the user. While TENS units work by blocking pain signals from reaching the brain, microcurrent units are thought to work by restoring normal electrical activity in the cells at the site of damage or injury. Microcurrent has been shown to actually stimulate tissue repair and improve circulation, so it has potential benefits that may go beyond short-term symptom control. Microcurrent treatment can be a little disconcerting at first, because it doesn't produce a sensation of its own like other types of electrical stimulation, so it's hard to know if it's doing anything (or even if the unit is on), until it begins to relieve symptoms.

Acupuncture

As with the acupressure methods discussed previously, acupuncture works with the flow and balance of energy through what are called meridians in the body. A meridian is not a structure per se, but a system of relay points for "wireless" communication in the body. There are several meridians in the body, most of which are named for organs they are associated with.

From a pain and symptom control standpoint, acupuncture works by changing the energy flow through the affected area. As with any treatment, it does not work for everyone, but it can be very effective and may be the only effective means of symptom control in some situations.

Many people have reservations about trying acupuncture, most often because of the fear of needles. Acupuncture needles are much thinner than injection needles, and in most cases are not particularly painful. Although there may be a mild sting or pinch when inserted, most people cannot feel them at all once they've been put in place. Even so, for those with a needle phobia, many acupuncturists practice at least one "needle-less" technique. These methods include acupressure (pressing or tapping on points as discussed earlier in this book), electrical point stimulation, laser point stimulation, and occasionally, heat, sound wave, and other types of point stimulation.

Many acupuncturists also practice other forms of Asian medicine and may recommend herbal remedies and/or specific diet or other lifestyle changes. These methods are intended to further re-balance the body's energy flow and enhance the effects of the acupuncture.

In most cases, spinal stenosis will require multiple sessions to get the best results from acupuncture, although many people get significant symptom improvement in the very first session.

Spinal Decompression

Spinal decompression (not to be confused with surgical decompression of the spine) is a form of traction. There are many spinal decompression devices on the market. The machines vary considerably in complexity and price, and this translates to wide ranges in treatment cost. There has been much controversy and debate regarding what actually qualifies as "true" spinal decompression (as opposed to regular spinal traction), and whether any of it is actually effective or not.

Overall, the studies regarding the effectiveness of spinal decompression are quite favorable. The basic concept of the treatment is that true spinal decompression uses a special computer-controlled motor to lull the body into a relaxed state so that the muscles do not resist the traction force (as much as is seen with traditional spinal traction). This allows the treatment to actually create negative pressure (suction) within the spinal discs, pulling in protruding disc material and improving hydration and nutrition to the disc to promote healing. In addition, like all traction, spinal decompression stretches soft tissue structures around the spine, and may reduce nerve compression caused by thickened ligament structures, as well as secondary muscular symptoms.

While all spinal decompression systems are traction machines of sorts, not all traction machines are able to produce decompressive forces sufficient to create a suction force (negative pressure) inside the spinal discs. As was discussed previously in this book, even regular traction is often beneficial for those with spinal stenosis, but actual spinal decompression systems can take things to a new level and often provide excellent long-term results, not just in relieving symptoms but in actually reducing the structural narrowing seen with some types of stenosis.

Generally, spinal decompression is done as a series of treatments performed over several weeks and periodic maintenance sessions are usually recommended at the completion of the initial series. It cannot be used in moderate to severe cases of stenosis due to bone spurring and overgrowth because the ragged edges of bone could potentially damage nerve structures during treatment. But for people with primarily disc and other soft-tissue related stenosis, it can be a very useful treatment.

Oral Prescription Medication

Medication is often the first line of treatment for people with spinal stenosis symptoms. Depending on the case, there are four main types of medication prescribed, and often two or more will be used at the same time. The primary down-side of any medication is potential side-effects, and the likelihood of significant side-effects increases the longer you are on a given medication, and with increasing numbers of different drugs being taken together. Whenever possible, it is best to use such medications only as a short-term symptom control measure, while other treatments that can potentially provide safer long-term management of the problem can be explored.

Anti-inflammatories are of course prescribed for the purpose of reducing inflammation and swelling that may be contributing to nerve compression. Prescription anti-inflammatory drugs may simply be a higher dose version of certain over-the counter NSAIDs (which were discussed previously), or they may be a different type of drug altogether.

One class of prescription anti-inflammatories that differs somewhat from over the counter drugs is the Cox-2 inhibitors such as Celebrex. Although Cox-2 inhibitors are themselves NSAIDs, they have a different mode of action from the usual over the counter varieties. Cox-2 inhibitors were initially thought to be more effective and safer than most other NSAIDS (which are Cox-1 inhibitors), but this has not proven to be the case. More recent research has indicated that Cox-2 inhibitor drugs are about the same in overall effectiveness to other NSAIDS, and there has been some indication that Cox-2 inhibitors can cause major cardiovascular side-effects in susceptible individuals. For this reason, the popularity of this class of drug has faded substantially among physicians in recent years.

Oral steroids are often prescribed in cases where inflammation plays a major role and these drugs typically have a stronger effect than NSAIDs. Unfortunately, that stronger effect comes at a price and oral steroids often produce significant side-effects, such as water retention, weight gain, mood swings, and decreased ability to fight off infections. In the short term, many people find these side-effects an acceptable trade-off for relief of their symptoms, but unless there simply is no other effective treatment, long-term use of these drugs is best avoided.

Pain relievers are drugs that reduce your conscious awareness of pain. They are potentially useful in times of severe symptoms, but because they dull the mind, they often fail to improve an individual's ability to carry out daily activities and may actually impair it. In addition, this type of drug tends to become less effective over time, requiring higher and higher doses for symptom relief and dependence/addiction are common issues with this group of drugs, especially when used long-term.

Muscle relaxers are intended to reduce muscle spasm and muscle contraction related symptoms; however, it has been the author's experience with patients taking these drugs that their effects on the muscles are minimal at best in most cases. Like pain relievers, muscle relaxers typically dull the mind and more often than not, it is this diminished consciousness that seems to actually provide the majority of whatever symptom relief muscle relaxers give, rather than a true relaxing effect on contracted muscles. As with pain relievers, muscle relaxers rarely improve a person's level of functioning, and problems with dependence and addiction are common.

"Nerve pain" drugs such as Lyrica and Gabapentin are relatively new entries in the treatment of spinal stenosis symptoms. The exact mode of action of these drugs is still unknown, and their effectiveness varies greatly from person to person. These types of drugs are generally considered to be a part of a long-term pain management strategy rather than a short-term method of symptom control; however, as with most drugs, they often gradually lose effectiveness over time and may require increasing doses to maintain results. The overall effectiveness short and long term and the side-effects of these drugs vary greatly. Some patients do quite well with them both short and long term, while others get essentially no symptom relief and/or suffer side-effects that are as bad or worse than the symptoms they are intended to treat. Still, because they potentially can provide good symptomatic relief, they are a reasonable option to try, particularly if other non-drug treatments have failed.

Invasive Treatments

Injections

There are several types of injectable medications used in treating spinal stenosis symptoms, but generally they fall into three categories: steroids, trigger point injections, and nerve blocks. Although all commonly-used injections are relatively safe for short-term symptom control, they do have risks (infections, allergic reactions, nerve damage from needle contact, etc.) and really are not good in and of themselves as a long-term treatment strategy - despite the fact that they are commonly used as such.

Steroid injections are commonly used for the purpose of reducing inflammation. Unlike oral steroids and other oral anti-inflammatories, steroid injections are targeted to the site of inflammation and typically have a stronger effect than orally-administered drugs. Of course, steroid injections provide the best results when inflammatory swelling is a major factor in symptoms, as opposed to cases when relatively severe disc protrusion, bone and ligament thickening, and other sources of direct narrowing of the spinal canals is present.

It is not unusual for steroid injections to initially increase symptoms, as the fluid volume of the injection itself can increase pressure around the nerves. Such increases in symptoms usually resolve within a day or so as the medication is absorbed by the tissues and it begins to lower inflammatory swelling.

The effectiveness of steroid injections varies greatly. Again, this likely has quite a bit to do with the relative contribution of inflammatory swelling to an individual's symptoms. For those who do get good results initially, the symptom relief is usually temporary and can last anywhere from a few days to a few years, but the relief in most cases lasts from a few weeks to a few months. Injectable steroids have the same potential side-effects as oral steroids (weight gain, mood swings, depressed immune function, etc.) but because of the concentrated dose near the spine, they present a greater risk of localized osteoporosis. A single round of steroid injections is unlikely to create significant bone thinning, but this side-effect is one reason why most doctors will limit the number of injections they give to an individual in a given period of time.

Although they do not correct any of the direct underlying causes of spinal stenosis symptoms, steroid injections can provide some relief for a while and can improve initial patient tolerance to exercises and other treatments which may provide a longer-term solution.

Trigger point injections are delivered to "knots" of muscle contraction that produce pain and other symptoms. Trigger points get their name from the fact that they often trigger referred pain and other symptoms some distance from the point of contraction. For example, certain trigger points in the buttock area can send symptoms down the leg that can mimic sciatica.

Various substances are used in trigger point injections, most commonly saline solution or some form of anaesthetic. In some cases, there is nothing injected at all – the needle is simply inserted into the point of contraction in what is known as "dry-needling". As you might have guessed from the last sentence, the effect of trigger point injections is thought by many to have more to do with the needle insertion into the contracted tissue than the substance being injected. As with massage techniques for trigger points, the purpose of trigger point injections is to relax the area of contraction to allow improved circulation and to stop the muscle from producing pain and referral symptoms.

Nerve blocks are injections of anaesthetic drugs onto or near irritated nerves for the purpose of blocking pain signals from those nerves to the central nervous system. This type of injection is usually reserved for chronic and treatment-resistant symptoms because they essentially "turn-off" the nerve for a time. This means that not only do they alleviate pain, but they also shut off most or all sensation from that nerve. This leaves the patient numb in the area the nerve supplies, and the lack of sensory information can interfere with normal activities and coordination. While in some cases, nerve blocks may be the best that can be done to manage spinal stenosis symptoms, they are not ideal and there are better long-term treatments for the majority of cases.

Surgery

Surgery is sometimes necessary to get lasting relief of spinal stenosis symptoms; however, there should be no rush to resort to surgical treatment before other methods have been exhausted. Although many people get excellent results from surgery, there are many who do not. Despite the fact that some people are statistically better candidates for surgery than others, there really is no way to fully predict in advance what the outcome of surgery will be for a given individual. A number of things can go wrong with any surgical procedure, and even when the procedure itself goes perfectly, post-surgical complications, such as scar tissue development, can result in a less than favorable long-term result.

Even when surgery is deemed to be appropriate, depending on the age and general condition of the patient, some surgeons will recommend delaying surgical procedures. Many of the causes of spinal stenosis can progress and/or recur after surgery, necessitating future surgeries. In general, subsequent surgeries tend to have less favorable outcomes and a greater incidence of complications. Delaying an initial surgery can sometimes minimize the need for subsequent surgeries and thereby reduces the potential for less than favorable long-term results.

Although symptoms can be difficult to tolerate, the only time surgery is really urgent and needs to be performed before conservative measures can be fully investigated is when "red-flag" symptoms of severe neurological compromise are present. These include severe muscle weakness in the legs and/or arms, loss of bowel and/or bladder function, and "saddle anaesthesia" (loss of sensation in the inner thighs and lower buttocks – the part of the body that would be in contact with a saddle when riding horseback). When these signs are present, surgical treatment is urgently needed to relieve pressure on nerves and should be done without delay in order to avoid permanent loss of function and disability.

There are several types of surgery that may be performed in spinal stenosis cases, and the type that is recommended all too often has as much or more to do with the surgeon(s) one consults, than your particular circumstances. Spine surgeons typically specialize in one or two types of procedures and a given surgeon will usually strongly favor his or her preferred technique(s) to anything else that may be appropriate and available for a given patient.

Asking a surgeon about other types of surgery (that he or she doesn't do) is kind of like asking the CEO of Ford Motor Company what he thinks about you buying a Toyota. Surgeons are human beings and like all of us, they have biases based on financial concerns and often plain old ego. For this reason, unless it is an emergency situation, the author recommends consulting with at least 3 different surgeons before deciding on which doctor you feel most comfortable with doing your surgery (if you decide to proceed with it at all after talking with the surgeons).

A common issue with any type of surgery is that surgeons often fail to explain the importance of exercises and preventive measures after surgery. All too often, the patient is released from care after the surgical wound is healed (and perhaps some weeks of physical rehabilitation) with no recommendations for how to keep their problems from returning over time. It is important to understand that while surgery can repair some of the existing damage, it usually does not correct the situations that caused the problem to develop in the first place, nor does it return the spine to a completely normal state. Taking good care of your spine by doing exercises and avoiding things that damage the spine are essential to avoiding a recurrence of problems months or years down the line. The exercises presented earlier in this book provide a good, easy to use program for prevention as well as for reducing symptoms when present.

The most common types of surgery for spinal stenosis are discussed below, with the more conservative techniques first. Whenever possible, the author recommends going with the most conservative method that is appropriate to the patient's situation. More conservative surgical approaches typically allow for faster recovery times and tend to have fewer post-surgical complications than more aggressive techniques. In addition, there is still usually much that can be done to improve things following a minimally invasive surgery that fails to get adequate results, but treatment options become severely limited following a fusion procedure when it doesn't work.

Minimally invasive surgery has several variations which may involve microsurgical tools, lasers, and other options, but the basic idea is the same for all of them. The surgeon makes small incisions and uses a scope to view the area being worked on as he or she trims away and uses suction to pull out excess disc, bone, and other tissue to open up the space in the nerve canals. In most cases, recovery from these procedures is pretty quick, with most patients able to resume the majority of their normal activities within a week or two. In addition to the fast initial recovery, minimally invasive procedures have much fewer problems with post-surgical scar tissue development than more aggressive surgical procedures.

There are cases in which minimally invasive surgery is not a good option. These include situations where there is structural instability in the spine, such as from torn ligaments or a condition known as spondylolisthesis (in which the back part of a vertebral bone is separated from the front and the weight-bearing part of the bone shifts forward).

The primary disadvantage of minimally invasive surgery is that because part of the wall of the disc may be trimmed away, it is sometimes left in a weakened state for some time after the surgery, making it susceptible to re-injury. In addition, when minimally invasive procedures are done in cases where there are multiple levels of the spine requiring work, it is not unusual for the surgeon to miss some significant problems, leaving some areas unaddressed and resulting in continued symptoms.

Spacer surgery is actually usually done as a minimally invasive procedure, but it bears mention separately because the purpose of this procedure is different than other minimally invasive surgeries. Rather than trimming away tissue that is narrowing the nerve canals, spacer surgery involves inserting a small spacer between the spinous processes (the bony projections that stick off the back of the vertebrae) of adjacent vertebrae to increase the space between them and in the intervertebral canals on each side of that level of the spine. To use an analogy, it's somewhat like propping a window open with a block of wood.

Spacer surgeries are usually quite effective initially, and they can work quite well long-term in some cases (in the author's experience, they tend to do best in older, more sedentary individuals). Unfortunately, the spacer does not appear to significantly prevent the progression of disc protrusions and posterior element stenosis, so ongoing progression of these problems can eventually necessitate further surgical intervention.

Laminectomy is a surgical procedure in which a portion of the back part of the bony arch of the vertebra is cut out and removed in order to open up space in the spinal canals. Laminectomy is somewhat more aggressive than minimally invasive techniques and requires larger incisions. This translates to a somewhat higher risk of infection and a greater tendency for post-surgical scar tissue development. Scar tissue can be a major problem in the months and years following the more aggressive types of surgery, as it sometimes grows into and around the spinal canals and nerves, resulting in spinal nerve compression and irritation of its own.

Although the author generally recommends minimally invasive procedures instead of laminectomy, there are situations where laminectomy may be preferable. In particular, cases where there are multiple adjacent levels of the spine with relatively severe stenosis, laminectomy may offer better long-term results.

Fusion surgery is sometimes done in combination with laminectomy. In a fusion, one or more of the spinal bones are joined together by either implanted bone chips (that eventually grow together) or more commonly by some sort of metal hardware. Although it is still a commonly-recommended procedure for all types of back pain and spinal stenosis, it is the author's opinion that fusion should be reserved for only cases where significant spinal instability has been diagnosed.

Instability is diagnosed by means of X-rays or motion imaging studies. Under normal circumstances, the spinal bones will retain pretty much the same front to back alignment with one another when you bend and move. When there is damage to the spinal ligaments, vertebral fracture, or when there is an unstable spondylolisthesis (not all spondylolistheses are significantly unstable), there may be a significant shift in the alignment of the spinal bones visible on X-rays taken in different positions (most commonly forward bending and backward bending), or on motion X-ray studies. In these cases, fusion is often necessary to eliminate the irritation caused by the instability.

Fusion is an aggressive form of surgery that involves relatively large incisions and it typically requires a long period (several months) of recovery. In addition to the greater risks presented by larger incisions and general anaesthesia for this type of procedure, it also tends to have the biggest problems with post-surgical scar tissue. The author recommends avoiding fusion surgery except when significant spinal instability is present or when all other treatment options have been exhausted.

Finally, although generally considered more of a pain-management technique than a type of surgery, in cases where all else has failed a surgically implanted electronic device may be installed in the spine. Somewhat similar to a TENS unit in concept, these devices known as dorsal column stimulators send electrical impulses directly into the spine via implanted electrodes to block pain signals from reaching the brain. Such devices are not universally effective and because of the cost and difficulties associated with them, they are usually considered a last resort for pain relief when all other methods have failed. They tend to be used primarily after surgical decompression techniques have already been attempted and in cases where severe neurological pain is the primary complaint (they do not help with losses of muscle function nor loss of sensation associated with spinal stenosis).

Conclusion

Although spinal stenosis can create significant challenges, in the vast majority of cases symptoms can be substantially improved or eliminated without surgery or other invasive treatments. The thing to bear in mind is that spinal stenosis is best thought of as a condition to be managed rather than something that can be "cured" once and for all. By finding effective treatment strategies and employing them not only to relieve symptoms but also as preventive measures, the majority of long-term problems associated with spinal stenosis can be avoided in most cases.

Review and Connect

I hope you have found this book helpful and if so, I ask that you consider posting a review on your favorite book retailer's website and/or any book review sites you enjoy.

For additional information, and/or if you have questions or comments regarding this book, I may be contacted via:

My website: http://www.AskDrBest.com/spinal-stenosis-book-resources

www.ingramcontent.com/pod-product-compliance
Lightning Source LLC
Chambersburg PA
CBHW080306290526

45790CB00005B/1947